a Consumer Publication

AVOIDING
HEART
TROUBLE

Consumers' Association
publishers of **Which?**
14 Buckingham Street
London WC2N 6DS

a Consumer Publication

edited by   Edith Rudinger

published by   Consumers' Association
publishers of Which?

Consumer Publications are
available from Consumers'
Association and from
booksellers. Details of other
Consumer Publications are
given at the end of this book.

Contents

Your heart and what it does   *page* 7
Heart rate   15
Blood pressure   18
What can go wrong   22
Abnormalities of rhythm   26
Valve disease   35
Heart failure   40
Angina pectoris   43
Coronary heart disease   48
Risk factors   49
Cigarette smoking   50
Raised blood pressure   61
Cholesterol and triglycerides   68
Stress   72
Physical inactivity   77
Men, women and heredity   80
Obesity and dietary factors   82
Oral contraceptives   87
Having a heart attack   89
Treatment after a heart attack   97
Rehabilitation   103
Glossary   111
Index   123

Your heart and what it does

The heart is a muscular pump designed to circulate blood around the body. For anyone not familiar with anatomy or biology, the whole set-up may be compared to a central heating system. The pump (heart) forces water (blood) under pressure (blood pressure) along the pipes (blood vessels: arteries) to all parts of the building (muscles, brain, kidneys, etc) where in the radiators (capillaries) heat (oxygen) is given off. The water then returns along more pipes (veins) to the pump (heart) from where it is sent to the boiler (lungs) to be reheated (oxygenated) and then back to the pump for recirculation.

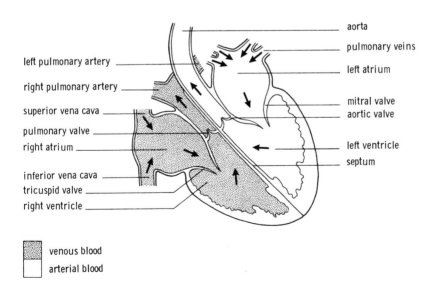

left pulmonary artery

right pulmonary artery

superior vena cava

pulmonary valve

right atrium

inferior vena cava

tricuspid valve

right ventricle

aorta

pulmonary veins

left atrium

mitral valve
aortic valve

left ventricle

septum

venous blood

arterial blood

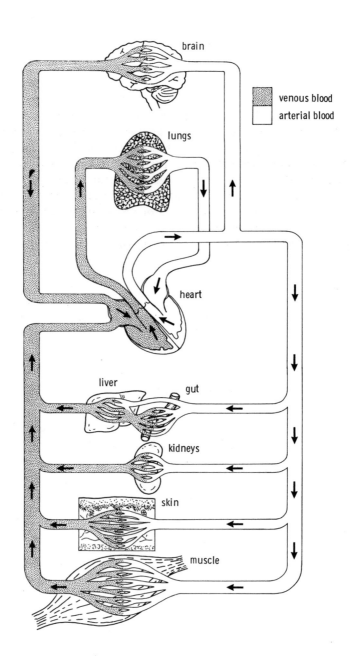

The heart is composed of two independent parts, a left and a right, joined together. Each has a receiving chamber (atrium) and a pumping chamber (ventricle). The left ventricle pumps blood into the main artery of the body (the aorta), and then into smaller and smaller branches (arterioles), down to the tiny blood vessels known as capillaries. Here, oxygen and nutrients are given off to the tissues and the waste gas carbon dioxide is taken up. The blood, which is now a purplish colour, then returns to the right part of the heart along veins, very small at first, then larger branches and finally the two big veins of the body (the venae cavae) into the right atrium. It then passes to the right ventricle which pumps it into the lungs. Here, the waste gas carbon dioxide is given off into the breath and oxygen absorbed from the breath. The oxygenated blood, now bright red in colour, flows into the left atrium; from there it passes to the left ventricle, to start the cycle over again.

There are valves between the two chambers in each half of the heart. The tricuspid valve separates the right atrium from the right ventricle; the mitral valve separates the left atrium from the left ventricle. The valves prevent blood being forced backwards along the way it has come. In other words, when blood has passed from the atria to the ventricles, these valves shut and only allow forward flow to the lungs and around the body.

There are also valves at the outlet of the right and left ventricle, known respectively as the pulmonary valve and aortic valve. After the ventricles have contracted and propelled their blood forwards, they relax, expand and fill up again with blood from their respective atria. At this time, the pulmonary and aortic valves close, in order to prevent blood which has just been pumped forward flowing back again into the ventricles.

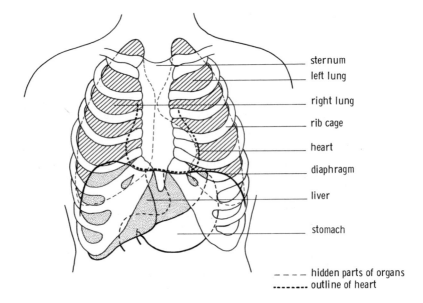

sternum
left lung
right lung
rib cage
heart
diaphragm
liver
stomach

_ _ _ _ hidden parts of organs
.... outline of heart

Lungs

The lungs are two elastic structures, one in each half of the chest on either side of the heart. They are designed for the interchange of gases (oxygen and carbon dioxide) between the air and blood. When we breathe in, the chest expands and the diaphragm, which is a thin sheet of muscle separating the chest from the abdomen, moves downwards. This reduces the pressure within the chest and the lungs expand. As they do so, air is sucked into them.

The lungs are composed of a vast number of minute air sacs (known as alveoli) which under the microscope appear a little like a sponge. The blood capillaries run very close to the alveoli, allowing gases to diffuse between air and blood.

During breathing out, the chest contracts, the diaphragm rises, the pressure within is increased and air is forced out.

The blood

Blood acquires its colour from the red blood cells which contain haemoglobin, a protein combined with iron-containing pigment. Haemoglobin is capable of combining with oxygen. When fully oxygenated, the blood is bright red in colour; when it has little or no oxygen, it is a purplish blue. Haemoglobin is capable of combining with carbon monoxide (a noxious gas found, for instance, in car exhaust fumes and cigarette smoke); when it does, this effectively prevents haemoglobin being available to combine with oxygen.

The blood also contains white blood cells and the very small cells concerned with blood clotting known as platelets, and carries many other substances, including the fats cholesterol and triglycerides, numerous nutrients, and waste products.

Blood vessels

Unlike the central heating water pipes, the blood vessels can dilate and contract, that is, make themselves wider or narrower. This is because a considerable part of the vessel walls is made of muscle, particularly in the arteries. When they narrow down, the amount of blood able to flow through them is reduced and when they widen, the amount is increased. As a result, some organs can receive a large flow and others a reduced one, in response to the need of the moment. For example, in cold weather, the vessels supplying the skin and underlying tissues constrict to reduce the blood flow and so reduce the loss of body heat—this accounts for the pale appearance of parts exposed to extreme cold. Another example is in physical exercise, when the blood flow to the muscles of the arms and legs is increased, in order to increase the supply of oxygen and other essential ingredients needed to satisfy the greater demand for energy.

Anatomy of main parts of circulation

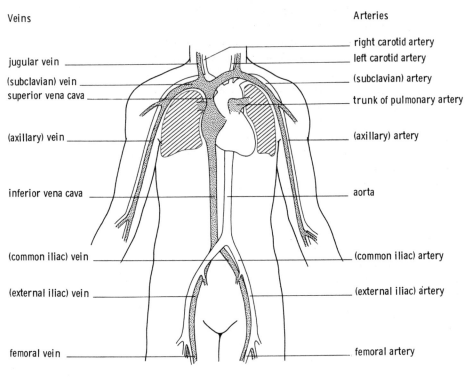

Veins

jugular vein

(subclavian) vein

superior vena cava

(axillary) vein

inferior vena cava

(common iliac) vein

(external iliac) vein

femoral vein

Arteries

right carotid artery

left carotid artery

(subclavian) artery

trunk of pulmonary artery

(axillary) artery

aorta

(common iliac) artery

(external iliac) artery

femoral artery

venous blood

arterial blood

Coronary arteries

The heart muscle, like any other muscle, has to have its own blood supply for the energy needed to make it work. This supply is not derived from the blood which is being pumped through the heart but is provided through arteries known as the coronary arteries, which encircle the heart like a crown.

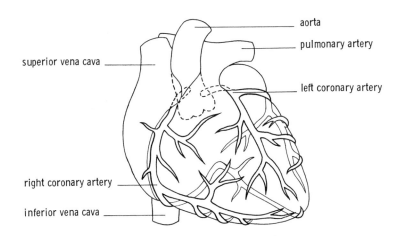

The left and right coronary arteries branch off the aorta into smaller and smaller vessels, in a similar way to those in other parts of the body, each supplying a part of the heart muscle. The blood finally returns into the right atrium via a system of veins draining into a large vein, the coronary venous sinus. It is vitally important for the proper functioning of the heart that the coronary arteries should be unobstructed.

A factor bringing about a narrowing of coronary arteries is the deposit of fatty and other materials (atheroma) in the lining of the arteries. The build-up of atheroma starts in youth and is an unavoidable part of ageing. It produces no symptoms until the narrowing is far advanced. Atherosclerosis, as this degenerative process is known, can affect arteries in all parts of the body and reduces the blood supply to the affected parts. The build-up can eventually block off the blood supply altogether.

lumen of artery

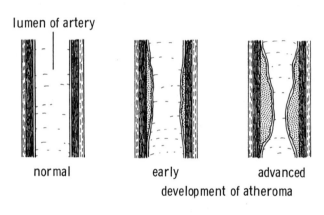

normal   early   advanced

development of atheroma

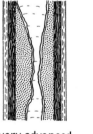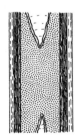

very advanced   occlusion

Electrical activation of the heart

The muscular contraction of the heart is set off by an electrical current developing in a very small piece of specialised tissue at the top of the right atrium. This excitation impulse passes downwards across both atria, causing them to contract and discharge their blood content into the right and left ventricles. By the time they have done this, the impulse has reached another piece of specialised tissue situated just at the top of the ventricles. After a short delay, which allows the atria to complete their contraction, the impulse is passed downwards to further specialised conducting fibres (a little like electrical wires) and from there to the muscles of the ventricles which then contract.

Heart rate

Each heart beat produces a pressure wave (pulse), transmitted down the arteries as blood is pumped into them from the left ventricle. Each pulse wave corresponds to a heart beat, but is felt over the radial artery at the wrist fractionally later, owing to the time taken for the pulse wave to travel to the wrist.

The normal pulse rate averages about 70 beats per minute. However, there is considerable variation between individuals, and also in any one person in different circumstances. The mere realisation that the pulse rate is being recorded may result in quite considerable speeding up, particularly in someone who is anxious.

Gentle physical activity, such as walking at a normal pace, is generally associated with a heart rate of about 80–100 beats a minute. More forceful exercise, such as hurrying up a couple of flights of stairs, may produce a heart rate of, say, 100–120 beats per minute. In general, the less fit the person, the higher the pulse rate for a given activity. A trained athlete may have a resting heart rate as low as 50 beats per minute, or even less, and would be exercising himself quite considerably before there is any substantial increase in his heart rate.

The maximum heart rate that can be reached by physical exercise varies with age: it is higher in the young and falls off with advancing age. For example, the maximum heart rate for a 20-year old man is around 190 per minute, for a 70-year old man, around 150 per minute.

An increased heart rate in response to physical exercise is normal. It is the way the body adapts to allow an increased amount of fuel to be supplied to muscles and organs and an increased amount of waste to be removed.

Nervous and chemical controls of heart rate

The central nervous system in the body is directly controlled by the conscious mind; but there is also an autonomic nervous system which is concerned with a variety of functions that go on independently of the will and of which we are largely unaware, such as digestion and the control of heart rate. This consists of two types of nerves, the sympathetic and parasympathetic, which have roughly opposite actions. The sympathetic nervous system acts through the intermediary of the two hormones noradrenaline and adrenaline. It is generally concerned with preparing the body for action, often referred to as preparing us for fight or flight. It increases the speed and force of the heart beat, thereby increasing the amount of blood circulating through appropriate parts, such as muscles, and so increasing the amount of oxygen and nutrients for chemical energy carried to them, and waste products removed.

The parasympathetic nervous system operates through a different chemical agent, acetylcholine. It slows the heart, diminishes its force of contraction and lowers the blood pressure, thus saving the heart from unnecessary fatigue. It also responds under certain circumstances to emotional stress and is the mechanism involved in the typical faint.

Emotional stress

The body responds to emotional stress as if it were physical stress: preparing a creature for fight or flight. In civilised man, neither action is very likely, so that the response, in terms of increase in heart rate, is, in fact, inappropriate. Perhaps primitive man did not have emotional hassles which did not also require the expenditure of physical energy.

The likely sequence of events might have been: man sees lion → increased stimulation by the sympathetic nervous system and increased adrenaline and noradrenaline release → increased heart rate → increased blood flow to vital organs and muscles → man equipped to grapple with lion or, if more sensible, to make a hasty retreat. The sequence of events in this day and age, however, is more like: man hears telephone ringing in office → intense business argument → increased sympathetic stimulation and adrenaline and noradrenaline release → increased heart rate → increased blood flow to muscles → man equipped to grapple physically with business opponent but does not do so, or at least not usually. And so an apparently wasted series of physiological events has occurred. The latent urge for some physical outlet is often externalised by fierce beating of the fist on the desk. (The restless pacing up and down of the expectant father is another example.)

Blood pressure

Blood pressure depends mainly on the force with which the left ventricle ejects blood into the arteries, the volume of blood ejected and the resistance to the flow within the arterial system, and is affected by the elasticity of the arteries themselves. It has two components: systolic pressure and diastolic pressure.

Systolic pressure is created as the left ventricle contracts and propels its blood content into the arteries. When the force of contraction increases, the pressure increases; and when it decreases, the pressure is reduced. Also, if the arteries narrow down, the systolic pressure increases—and vice versa. This phenomenon is similar to the effect of putting a thumb over a running water tap. The more the outlet is narrowed, the greater the force with which the water jet comes out.

Diastolic pressure is the pressure in the arterial system while the left ventricle relaxes and refills with blood in preparation for its next beat. It is determined by the relationship between the size and condition of the arteries and the volume of blood in them. The blood volume is more or less constant under normal resting conditions. The major factor affecting diastolic pressure is therefore the calibre of the arterial system, and the elasticity of the muscle in the walls of the blood vessels.

If the smaller arteries lose their elasticity, as the result of ageing or of disease, they cannot so readily accommodate what the heart ejects and the pressure rises—the systolic much more than the diastolic.

Raised blood pressure is known as hypertension. It may affect the systolic blood pressure alone, occasionally the diastolic pressure alone, or both together.

Measuring blood pressure

Blood pressure is measured by a sphygmomanometer. This consists of an inflatable cuff, placed round the person's upper arm, connected to a pressure gauge which contains a column of mercury and to a hand pump with which air is pumped into the cuff. As the pressure of air in the cuff is increased, the mercury rises up the column and the artery in the arm is constricted. The doctor or nurse uses a stethoscope placed over the artery at the elbow to listen to the pulse. When the artery is fully compressed, no pulse can be heard, or felt at the wrist.

When air is slowly released from the cuff, the pressure and the column of mercury fall. At the point when blood starts to flow again through the compressed artery, the pulse can be heard, or felt, and the level of mercury at this point is read. This reading gives the systolic blood pressure.

As the pressure falls lower, at a certain point a change in the sound of the pulse can be recognised, and at this point the diastolic pressure can be read.

Blood pressure is usually expressed in millimetres (mm) of mercury (Hg) as a ratio of systolic to diastolic, for example 120/80 mmHg. In some countries it is expressed in centimetres: 12/8 cmHg.

The person most likely to take your blood pressure is your GP, either because he suspects you have a raised blood pressure or during a medical examination for some other cause.

The most useful blood pressure reading is obtained when your body is resting and you are relaxed. Hurry or worry is likely to raise your blood pressure. A person who is worried about the visit to the surgery and who has had a hectic rush arriving on time, may have an initial figure which is high. Your GP may repeat the measurement at the end of the consultation if you have become more relaxed. But if someone is very anxious about the consultation, resting may not lower the measurement. You may be asked to come again on later occasions to have your blood pressure taken.

Your blood pressure may also be taken on other occasions such as at your place of work by the medical officer, at an ante-natal or family planning clinic, or in a hospital.

Visiting a hospital, for people who are not used to it, can produce a rise in blood pressure, and anxiety can make this worse. Sometimes a person seen in an outpatient department is told that he has high blood pressure and advised to go and see his GP about it, and is then surprised—and not always completely reassured—when told by the GP that his blood pressure is normal.

Raised blood pressure

There is no exact threshold at which pressure ceases to be normal, nor exact levels at which hypertension is mild, moderate or gross. A rough and somewhat arbitrary description would be:

systolic pressure
between 150 and 180 mmHg = mild hypertension
between 180 and 210 mmHg = moderate hypertension
between 210 and 240 mmHg = severe hypertension
between 240 and 300 mmHg = gross hypertension

diastolic pressure
between   95 and 110 mmHg = mild hypertension
between 110 and 125 mmHg = moderate hypertension
between 125 and 140 mmHg = severe hypertension
above   140 mmHg   = gross hypertension

However, such classifications are artificial and have a limited use-
fulness from anything but the purely descriptive point of view, particularly with mild and moderate hypertension. There is no hard and
fast cut-off point below which there is no risk of complications and
above which there is a risk. Rather, there is a relative degree of risk
on a sliding scale from mild hypertension upwards, with the risk
increasing progressively. The higher the pressure, the more likely
there is trouble ahead.

What can go wrong

Symptoms of heart trouble include shortness of breath, faintness, palpitations, swelling of ankles. But any of these may be due to non-cardiac causes, such as anaemia, bronchitis, varicose veins—or anxiety. Go and see your doctor with any such symptoms, if only to be reassured.

Chest pain may be caused by indigestion; by incipient shingles where pain precedes the rash by about a week; by fibrositis in the muscles between the ribs; by arthritis in the neck and chest vertebrae; by stomach ulcers and hiatus hernia; by pleurisy and by pneumonia. So, any chest pain may be a sign of serious disease. Do not pretend to yourself that it is just indigestion, but go and consult your doctor. Also, any attacks of unconsciousness should certainly be reported to the doctor.

Unlike the theatrical demonstration of pain from the heart, when the actor clutches his left breast (where he thinks his heart is), true heart muscle pain tends to occur in the centre of the chest.

Unexplained chest pains

Many people develop pains in the chest which to them, but much less often to their doctor, seem to come from the heart muscle. Some of these pains have an easily detected and understandable organic cause; or the pain may be muscular in nature, sometimes associated with prolonged stress.

Pains in the chest that are due to causes which, although ill-understood, are thought not to involve any disease of the heart, have been labelled effort syndrome and cardiac neurosis. These pains tend most frequently to occur in anxious or introspective individuals, but to label them imaginary would be both unkind and unfair. The pains tend to be stabbing, or sometimes aching. They may occur at rest; if brought on by exertion, they usually persist for a fairly long time even when the sufferer rests.

Anyone with unexplained pains in the chest should see the doctor. Do not try to make your own diagnosis, particularly in so important a matter as the heart. Even at the risk of feeling embarrassed at seeming to waste the doctor's time, go to him and describe your symptoms. A good doctor would rather see a patient even if all that is needed is reassurance, than let a genuine organic problem go untreated. Most general practitioners can distinguish false from genuine angina, and can reassure the sufferer accordingly—and in most instances nothing more is required. In cases of doubt, the general practitioner will refer you to the expertise of a cardiologist.

Outpatient examination

What happens at an outpatient heart clinic depends on the particular hospital or unit. Your medical history will be taken and the cardiologist may ask you some of the same questions as the general practitioner did. He may carry out some of the same physical examinations plus some other tests, and may send you to another part of the hospital for a chest X-ray or blood test.

Blood tests may show high levels of the two main fats in the blood, cholesterol and triglycerides, which may predispose to the development of coronary heart disease. Also, unsuspected diabetes may be detected by blood glucose analysis and analysis of urine. A blood test is usually done in the morning, after a 12–14 hour fast. A small amount of blood is taken from a vein, for analysis.

The chest X-ray may reveal an enlargement of the heart, or an abnormality in its shape or abnormalities of major blood vessels.

Physical examination

You must tell the doctor of any symptoms that you think are relevant, and even those that may not be. Physical examination is likely to include

○ taking blood pressure readings;

○ examination of the pulse for rate, rhythm and quality, including pulses in the arms and legs and neck;

○ inspection of veins in the neck for over-distension (which might be a sign of fluid retention and possible right-sided heart failure);

○ feeling the heart beat on the chest wall to determine the overall size of the heart and the quality of the beat (an abnormal feel of the heart beat against the chest can indicate an enlarged heart);

○ examination of the eyes with an ophthalmoscope (for changes in the blood vessels);

○ listening to the heart with a stethoscope to detect murmurs (possibly caused by faulty heart valves) or other abnormal sounds;

○ feeling the abdomen to detect possible liver enlargement;

○ inspecting the ankles for swelling (which may be associated with right-sided heart failure).

ECG

The electrocardiogram is one of the mainstays of cardiological tests. As part of any investigation into heart trouble, a reading of your heart beat will be made with the help of an electrocardiograph. This is a machine which is connected to the patient by one set of wires attached to each arm and each leg and one or more connecting wires placed onto different parts of the chest. It is impossible to get a shock because it is the electricity already in you that is being recorded, not a current flow conducted into the body. The whole process takes only a few minutes. There is no discomfort, you merely have to lie down and keep as relaxed and as still as possible. (Some GPs have a portable battery-operated ECG machine which can be taken to a patient's home.)

As the electrical activation of the heart proceeds, current travels to the surface of the body and can be recorded by electrodes at the end of the wires placed on the limbs and chest.

Each heart beat produces a wave pattern which the doctor can then assess as being normal or abnormal. It is the spread of the excitation wave across the heart which produces the electrocardiogram figure.

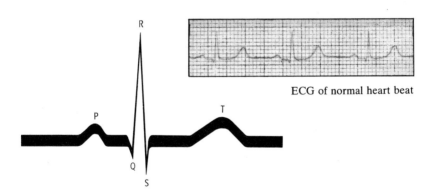

ECG of normal heart beat

P = electrical activation of atrium
QRS = electrical activation of ventricles
T = recharging of ventricles

An electrocardiogram is particularly useful in detecting rhythm disturbances.

Abnormalities of heart rhythm

Probably the commonest abnormality of heart rhythm consists of ectopic beats (the word ectopic means displaced, out of place).

Ectopic beats arise when the electrical excitation develops in a different part of the heart from the normal and a beat occurs sooner than it should; there is then a correspondingly slightly longer rest before the next beat. Ectopic beats arising in the atria are not very dissimilar from the normal beat. Those arising in the ventricles, however, activate the heart in a different direction, and those arising at the bottom or apex of the ventricle virtually result in a completely reversed path. (They produce a totally different wave form on the electrocardiogram.) The person is often unaware of any except the ventricular ectopic beats which may give rise to palpitations. Palpitation is defined as an awareness of the heart beat, and has a variety of forms. With ectopic beats, people usually describe a sensation of a bump in the chest or the throat, as if their heart is 'jumping', 'missing' or 'skipping' a beat. It is the beat after the ectopic beat that causes this sensation; the increased gap between the ectopic and subsequent normal beat increases the length of time during which the heart fills with blood. This increases the stretch on the heart muscle which then responds by an increased force of contraction— so that you become aware of it.

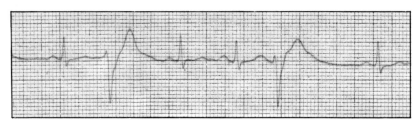

ventricular ectopic

Occasional ectopic beats are considered normal. In general, those arising in the atria tend to be of less importance than those arising in the ventricles, and you are also less likely to be aware of them. Ventricular ectopic beats occurring more frequently than say 6 per minute may be associated with underlying heart disease. On the other hand, they may be entirely due to, or at least made worse by, too much alcohol, tobacco, tea, coffee or cocoa, and by stress. Irregular heart beats may be unpleasant and alarming but are not in themselves dangerous, and do not necessarily lead to the development of abnormal functioning of the heart.

attacks of abnormally fast heart rate (paroxysmal tachycardia)

When the abnormal initiation of the heart beat takes over completely, and results in a continued series of ectopic beats, the person may feel that the heart suddenly starts to race. The beginning and end of such a paroxysm or attack is like the turning on and off of a switch. The attack is characterised by coming on and ending very suddenly; it may last a few seconds or minutes or even hours. In ventricular tachycardia, the disordered sequence of activation interferes with the efficient filling of the chambers and contraction, so that the person may feel weak, breathless, incapacitated, needing to sit down and stop whatever he is doing at the time.

In a heart which is already damaged, such an attack may lead to more serious abnormality of rhythm, or may result in heart failure. In an otherwise healthy heart, however, attacks may pass off with little or no residual disability.

irregular impulses (atrial fibrillation)

When the sequence of activation becomes completely disorganised and multiple points of activation develop in the atria, less blood gets into the ventricles so that less blood is pumped out with each beat. The atria do not empty themselves in normal regular contractions, the ventricles beat irregularly, sometimes rapidly. The combination results in about a 15 per cent drop in efficiency. The person has a disagreeable sensation in the chest, associated with a general feeling of being unwell. In a heart which is already acting less efficiently for other reasons, this reduction of 15 per cent in the amount of blood pumped out at each beat may be important.

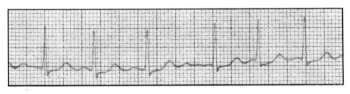

atrial fibrillation

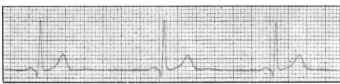

bradycardia

slow heart beat (bradycardia)

Bradycardia is defined as a heart rate below 60 beats per minute. In a healthy young person, and especially a trained athlete, this is quite normal and needs no treatment. However, in an elderly person, a sudden development of bradycardia, especially if accompanied by a feeling of faintness, deserves further investigation and possibly treatment. The slow rate may lead to the development of more serious abnormalities of rhythm.

heart block

If the normal electrical activation of the heart is blocked, through whatever cause, the ventricles may beat on their own initiative at about 40 beats per minute. This may cause hardly any symptoms, particularly if the rate is fairly steady. But if the rate drops considerably below 40, this may result in fainting, owing to inadequate blood flow to the brain. Any attacks of unconsciousness should certainly be reported to the doctor.

Treatment for irregularities of heart rate and rhythm

An increasingly wide variety of drugs is available, both for the prevention of paroxysmal attacks and for treatment of an acute attack itself. Many of these drugs that regulate the heart action have unpleasant side effects, of which the doctor should warn you.

Amongst the drugs commonly used for the treatment of rhythm disturbances are the beta-blocking agents; also digitalis, quinidine, procainamide, mexiletine, verapamil, and a number of others. The instructions about the use of the drugs have to come from the general practitioner or the hospital consultant. Report any severe side effects, in case a change in prescription or dosage will help.

electronic pacemakers

A patient with severe bradycardia may be given a pacemaker. A pacemaker consists of an electrode on the end of a wire inserted into the heart (usually the right ventricle).Impulses sent along the wire from a small electronic box cause the heart muscle to contract, and initiate or regulate the heart beat.

A fixed-rate pacemaker will put impulses into the heart at a pre-set rate and fire continuously at that rate. A demand pacemaker is set for a certain heart rate and only fires if the patient's own heart rate falls below this.

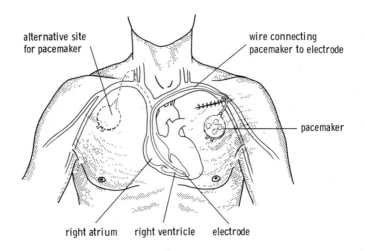

alternative site for pacemaker

wire connecting pacemaker to electrode

pacemaker

right atrium   right ventricle   electrode

The electronic box which produces the current is situated by the side of the patient's bed in a hospital; or, for permanant pacing, a miniaturised version is implanted, generally underneath the skin near the armpit. The pacemaker box may be inserted in other positions, such as in the abdominal wall—particularly in children or a very thin adult—where it would cause less obvious stretch on the skin and is preferable cosmetically.

The battery life of the pacemaker units used to be limited to about 2–3 years; nowadays they last for at least 5 years and even up to 15 years. But checks have to be made on the state of the batteries; this entails regular follow-up visits to the pacemaker clinic in a hospital.

A person with a permanent pacemaker can lead a fully normal life. But pacemakers may be affected not only by the anti-theft checkouts of libraries, about which there is usually a warning, but also the airways security screening doorways.

Other uses of ECG

An electrocardiogram may also show features suggesting any thickening of the heart muscle not yet apparent clinically or on X-ray. An ECG can help to detect the presence of coronary disease before symptoms appear, and can even show up undue reaction to stress.

24-hour monitoring
Devices are available for making a 24-hour electrocardiogram. Two, three, or four electrodes are stuck to the person's chest, connected by a fine cable to a miniaturised recorder which records the electrocardiogram over a period of up to 24 hours onto a magnetic tape, which can then be analysed. The recorder is carried on the person inside a pocket or strapped around the waist. The apparatus usually incorporates an event-marker so that as and when symptoms occur, the patient can press a button which identifies the event on the recording tape.

Blood pressure, too, can be similarly recorded for 24 hours. For this, however, a thin tube has to be inserted into an artery.

These 24-hour monitoring devices for ECG are not available in all hospitals, but are used fairly generally in teaching hospitals.

exercise test
Although an electrocardiogram, taken when the person is at rest, is an important part of routine screening, it has limitations. To some extent, the ECG tends to reflect what happened in the past and can show up that a mild heart attack has taken place in the past. But a normal ECG trace does not mean that you will be free of heart trouble in the future. In a number of people who have angina, or symptomless coronary disease, the resting ECG trace is normal.

An electrocardiogram obtained during an exercise test, in which stress is applied to the heart, can record the present position and at the same time offer a prediction of future events.

In good hands, this test is safe and informative but done casually it can be dangerous and misleading. It is carried out on a static bicycle or, preferably, on a treadmill. Electrodes are placed on the person's chest, connected by a cable to the recording equipment. The subject starts at a fairly low workload and increases progressively until he stops because of fatigue, breathlessness, chest pain or other symptoms, or the test is stopped by an operator because of changes in the electrocardiographic wave form or changes in blood pressure.

A treadmill exercise test carried out to the patient's comfortable limit of endurance (or to the attainment of a target heart rate) is about 70 per cent accurate in detecting latent coronary disease. However, about 10 per cent of people whose exercise-test electrocardiogram appears to suggest that they will have heart trouble within the next 5 years, in fact never do.

Echocardiography

Echocardiography is an investigative technique which involves bouncing sound waves through the chest in order to map out the shape of the structures within it; a similar procedure is fairly widely used in obstetrics. The technique is also known as ultra-sound.

This technique makes it possible for abnormalities of valves to be detected, also abnormalities of thickness of muscle, and of the way the muscle contracts. Echocardiography can also detect less common problems such as fluids collecting around the heart, or a tumour within the heart.

Echocardiography is performed with the patient lying half on his back, half on his left side, on a couch; no needles, tubes or anything else are inserted into the body. A recording is made by placing a sensor, which is about the size and shape of a ballpoint pen, on the patient's chest and positioning it at various angles. The process takes about 15 minutes to half an hour, during which time the patient has to lie as still as is reasonably possible, but he may be asked to vary his position very slightly from time to time during the recording.

At present, echocardiography is carried out only when there are special indications as a result of other examinations and tests. Teaching hospitals and many of the larger district general hospitals have facilities for echocardiography. The equipment is very expensive and considerable technical skill is required to make the recording and to interpret the findings.

Cardiac catheterisation

Cardiac catheterisation is in no way a routine test, but a highly specialised technique for which particular skills and equipment are required. Tubes are inserted into an artery and/or vein, either in the arm or leg, and passed into particular parts of the heart, as required. Through these tubes, blood samples may be taken, pressures recorded or radio-opaque dyes injected so that cine X-rays may be taken.

Cardiac catheterisation is usually done with local anaesthesia so that the catheter can be inserted through the skin without causing pain.

It is becoming common practice for the patient to come into hospital in the morning, as a day patient, have the investigation, and leave hospital later the same day. Some centres prefer the patient to be in hospital for at least the subsequent night, in case there are any complications, such as transient disturbances of heart rhythm, or oozing from the wound.

One of the commoner uses for cardiac catheterisation is coronary angiography. A catheter is passed into the opening of the coronary artery, and radio-opaque dye is injected which shows up on cine X-rays. This allows the anatomy of the coronary arteries to be fairly accurately shown, so that areas of narrowing or complete blockage can be detected. The doctors can thus assess whether surgery is feasible and would be helpful. Usually, dye is also injected into the left ventricular cavity, and recorded on cine X-rays to show up the pattern of contraction. This, too, helps to decide whether the person is suitable for surgery. Angiography is also a useful procedure for detecting narrowing or incompetence of valves.

Valve disease

The valves separating the right and left atria from their respective ventricles are the tricuspid and mitral valves; those at the outlet of the right and left ventricles are the pulmonary and aortic valves.

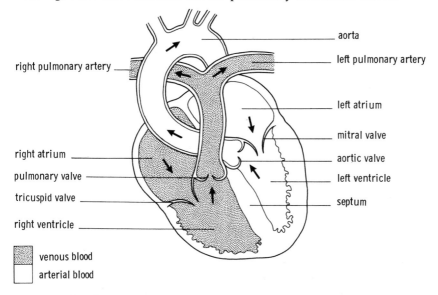

right pulmonary artery

aorta

left pulmonary artery

left atrium

mitral valve

right atrium

aortic valve

pulmonary valve

left ventricle

tricuspid valve

septum

right ventricle

venous blood

arterial blood

narrowed valves
Narrowed (stenosed) valves may be congenital (that is, the person was born with the defect) or acquired as a result of damage from, for instance, rheumatic fever; or narrowing may develop because of a sclerosing process, that is, a gradual loss of elasticity.

Stenosis of the mitral valve or the tricuspid valve hinders the forward flow of blood from their respective atria to the ventricles; stenosis of the pulmonary valve hinders the forward flow of blood from the right ventricle to the lungs.

Stenosis of the aortic valve reduces the amount of blood that is pumped around the body with each contraction. Whereas this may be adequate at rest, it may become insufficient when increased demands are placed on the heart (such as during physical exercise)—and symptoms such as fainting may result.

incompetent valves
If valves fail to provide an adequate seal and therefore leak, they are known as incompetent or regurgitant valves. Incompetence of the pulmonary and aortic valves allows blood to flow back from the arteries into the ventricles. If the tricuspid and mitral valves do not close properly, blood can regurgitate back from the ventricles to the atria.

A leaking aortic valve allows part of the expelled blood to return to the left ventricle where it mixes with the incoming blood from the left atrium. This throws an increased load on the ventricle and results in dilatation, and eventually in heart failure. The main symptoms of aortic regurgitation are breathlessness—difficulty in breathing when lying flat and sudden attacks of intense shortness of breath, particularly at night.

The valves most commonly affected are those on the left-hand side of the heart (mitral and aortic valves). Disease of the mitral valve results in a backward pressure on the lungs; the blockage to blood entering the left ventricle prevents blood leaving the lungs. As a result of the back pressure in the blood vessels in the lungs, some of the fluid extrudes from the capillaries into the lung substance itself. This produces a water-logging effect, the symptom of which is shortness of breath.

Valve disease (either regurgitation or narrowing) can lead to what is popularly known as an enlarged heart, caused by thickening of the heart muscle in response to the extra strain and by the compensatory dilatation of the chamber to cope with the extra blood brought back into it.

Either incompetence or narrowing, if sufficiently severe, may result in heart failure.

infection
Damaged heart valves are peculiarly susceptible to becoming infected; the condition is known as sub-acute bacterial endocarditis. It is difficult to get rid of and can lead to death despite full antibiotic treatment. It may turn a relatively trivial lesion into a life-destroying one in a very short time.

A variety of micro-organisms may be responsible; amongst those most likely to cause the infection is the streptococcus viridans which normally inhabits the mouth without causing symptoms, and organisms that normally inhabit the gastro-intestinal tract. Neither dentistry nor any endoscopic procedures of the gastro-intestinal tract should be carried out without antibiotics on a person with this condition. Any patient with a defective heart valve should tell the dentist about it; most hospital clinics provide a special card, warning both the patient and the dentist.

other dangers
People with certain forms of valve disease, particularly mitral valve disease associated with atrial fibrillation, are prone to develop blood clots in the left atrium. The clots may then pass into the left ventricle and out into the bloodstream, ending up in the small peripheral blood vessels where they can cause an obstruction (embolism) and subsequent death of the part of the tissue normally served by that artery beyond the clot. An embolism can end up in the kidneys, limbs, spleen, eyes—or the brain, causing a stroke.

Because of the risk of blood clots developing, anti-coagulant treatment is usually given, on a long-term basis. The anti-coagulant dosage has to be monitored regularly to maintain the right level of blood clotting power. (Too little clotting ability can result in internal bleeding.) This requires regular visits, generally not less frequently than once a month, to a clinic or the GP, even if this is inconvenient or difficult for the patient.

rheumatic heart disease
Rheumatic heart disease which was a major problem in the earlier part of this century is now much less common in the United Kingdom. The exact nature of the disease is not totally clear; it is considered to be an abnormal tissue response in people who are sensitised to infection by the beta haemolytic streptococcal organism. It usually tends to occur some weeks after an infection by this organism (often a throat infection) and occurs most commonly in childhood and early adult life. In the nowadays rare cases of rheumatic fever in a child, the child may have to remain on penicillin treatment until he is in his twenties.

Rheumatic fever tends to affect the valves of the heart, particularly the mitral valve. Once the intitial damage has been done, there generally tends to follow a latent period of some years before the slow progressive deterioration leads to symptoms.

surgery for valve disease

Where one of the valves has become abnormally narrowed, an operation called a valvotomy can be carried out during which a special dilating instrument is inserted and opened rather like an umbrella, forcing the valvular opening to widen. During the operation, the heart continues to function normally.

In most other cardiac operations, blood is taken from the right side of the heart, oxygenated through a special 'heart-lung' machine and re-pumped into the arteries so that the heart can be opened, valves removed and artificial ones put in their place, or any other defects repaired, while the heart is stopped but all vital organs are supplied with blood.

In all but the most complex and advanced cases, the replacement of damaged valves has now become a relatively risk-free procedure.

The old valve is usually cut out and replaced by one taken from a dead human heart (homograft) or from another species of animal, such as a pig (heterograft). Artificial valves made from a variety of synthetic materials are also available; hospitals can stock a complete range of sizes, so that a correct fit is always available. The disadvantage of artificial valves is that they generally require permanent anti-coagulant treatment afterwards, to prevent blood clots forming which become a potential source of embolism.

Heart failure

Heart failure sounds frightening—and if it occurs suddenly, it is frightening. However, it does not mean that the heart fails completely, but that its ability to pump blood around the body is impaired.

Heart failure ranges in degree from mild, when the heart fails to pump adequately and causes little distress, to severe heart failure which may be life threatening.

Someone who has been very active during the day, especially a person with high blood pressure, may be woken from sleep by extreme breathlessness, wheezing and coughing due to sudden heart failure. An attack of this nature requires urgent medical help.

Generally, however, heart failure develops slowly. The first signs include shortness of breath, a feeling of fatigue, swelling of the ankles which gets more pronounced as the day wears on and eventually difficulty in breathing when lying flat in bed at night.

left heart failure
This occurs when the left ventricle is unable to pump out an adequate amount of blood into the aorta and around the body. It may occur for instance when part of the heart muscle of the left ventricle receives an insufficient supply of blood because the coronary arteries are narrowed, or when part of the muscle has been damaged by a heart attack.

Alternatively, the ventricle may have outgrown its own blood supply. This may happen when the ventricle thickens in response to the extra effort involved in pumping out its contents against the resistance of a narrowed aortic valve. Or the muscle may be enlarged for no known reason or may be damaged by toxic agents such as alcohol or by germ infection.

The heart may also fail if there is an obstruction between the left atrium and the left ventricle, for instance a narrowed mitral valve, so that the ventricle cannot fill properly, or if blood is allowed to escape backwards into the left atrium owing to incompetence of the mitral valve.

Left heart failure leads to two sets of problems, those in front and those behind. The 'forward' problems are created by inadequate blood flow to vital organs such as the brain and kidneys, which may result in faintness and in salt and water retention by the kidneys. The 'backward' problems are concerned with the lungs. Despite left side failure, the right ventricle may continue to pump its blood efficiently into the lungs. But because the failing left side of the heart is unable to deal with the incoming flow of blood, there is a hold-up and the lungs become congested with blood. The excess amount of blood in the vessels within the lungs seeps out as fluid into the lung substance. When the air sacs become waterlogged and cannot take in air, this causes wheezy, laboured breathing in the person.

right heart failure
The majority of the problems that afflict the heart tend to affect the left half. Right heart failure is much less common on its own. The right ventricle has less work to do than the left, pumping its blood out into the lungs at a pressure of about 20 mmHg, as against 120 mmHg, or more, in the case of the left ventricle.

It is less often damaged by coronary artery disease, possibly because being thinner and under relatively low pressure it is more easily perfused with blood even if the coronary artery supply is reduced.

But there are some situations in which the right ventricle may fail, for instance when the outflow of blood to the lungs is obstructed, imposing more work on the right ventricle. This may be caused by a narrowed pulmonary valve, or the small pulmonary arteries may offer increased resistance through them (perhaps as a result of long standing bronchitis or other lung disease).

The breathlessness caused by right heart failure is much less than in the case of left-sided failure, but a back pressure may affect the venous system, causing distension of the veins. This (particularly if there is reduced blood flow to vital organs such as the kidneys) may result in fluid accumulation in the body and cause swelling of the ankles (oedema), enlargement of the liver and sometimes distension of the abdomen.

combined heart failure
When the right ventricle fails as a consequence of the resistance imposed on it by the left ventricle failing to clear the flow, a combined failure of left and right heart results. This type of congestive heart failure has the features of both left and right heart failure: congestion of the lungs behind a failing left side of the heart, and enlargement of liver and swelling of ankles behind a failing right side.

treatment
Medical treatment for heart failure includes the administration of drugs to clear the excess fluid retention (diuretics) and drugs such as digoxin to increase the strength of the heart beat. In the case of left heart failure, the doctor will advise the patient to avoid lying flat and to sleep propped up because this has an important effect on the blood distribution between body and lungs.

Angina pectoris

Angina is pain from the heart muscle itself. It often extends up to the neck and down the left arm and may be felt in the region over the stomach. It is of a gripping or choking nature and often associated with a sensation of breathlessness and a tendency to acute anxiety.

Angina is triggered off by a disparity between oxygen supply and oxygen demand. The exact physiological mechanism is still not fully understood. When narrowing of the coronary arteries reduces the blood flow to the heart muscle, the blood supply may remain sufficient for the demand of the heart under tranquil resting conditions. But when an extra load is put on it, such as by physical exercise, the supply may become insufficient and angina result. When there is no longer an extra demand, so that the blood supply is again adequate, the pain starts to disappear.

Anginal pain is distinguished from other chest pains because it is brought on by effort, particularly after a meal or on going out in the cold, or by emotional stress, and is quickly relieved by rest or relaxation.

Emotion is probably a less common precipitating factor than effort. Emotion results in an increased release of adrenaline and noradrenaline into the bloodstream, both of which increase the oxygen requirement of the heart muscle. If the coronary arteries are partially obstructed, the blood supply to the heart muscle may therefore be insufficient and angina result.

Narrowing of the aortic valve, too, may produce angina on exertion, particularly if the heart muscle is thickened as a result of the faulty valve.

The pain of angina is probably produced because of some form of accumulation of waste products resulting from the disparity between oxygen supply and oxygen demand.

Treatment of angina

First and foremost, identify—and avoid—situations likely to bring on an attack.

Anyone with angina should examine his or her life-style and pay attention to general factors such as cigarette smoking (absolutely forbidden) and excess weight (to be reduced). The person should get adequate sleep, try to avoid overwork and becoming overtired, and allow time for hobbies, relaxation, and holidays. If possible, the standard of physical fitness should be increased by gradually increasing the amount of exercise taken. Such training helps to reduce the sudden rise in heart rate produced by exercise in an untrained person. But violent exercise is dangerous and should be avoided.

Gradually increasing exercise, short of bringing on angina, can sometimes be very beneficial. The reason may be that exercise encourages the growth of collateral blood vessels. Where one or other of the larger coronary arteries is partially or totally blocked, other smaller vessels may grow larger to do some of the work of the blocked artery. Another possibility may be that exercise, by improving general muscle tone, improves the blood flow to muscles and the removal of waste products from muscles throughout the body, so that the workload on the heart is reduced and the angina lessened.

drugs for angina

Drug therapy has transformed the life of many angina sufferers. Glyceryl trinitrate (trinitrin, or GTN—sometimes erroneously called TNT) is a useful and highly effective drug to cut short an attack of pain, or to prevent one altogether by taking a tablet before exercise or other situations which are known to bring on the pain, such as hurrying to catch a train. The tablets should therefore be carried on the person (or kept beside the bed at night) to have ready for use at all times. A small stoppered container should be used to keep them airtight, otherwise they lose their effect. When they are fresh, they produce a slight tingling sensation in the mouth.

The tablets should be bitten into two or three pieces and placed under the tongue so that they can dissolve in the mouth, rather than be swallowed: they are absorbed directly into the bloodstream. The effect is to dilate the blood vessels; it takes about two minutes for the tablets to work. The side effects may include palpitations, dizziness and headache. If they are very troublesome, report them to the doctor: there are half-strength tablets available.

Apart from GTN which acts on the blood vessels, beta-blocking drugs are prescribed for angina sufferers. Beta-blocking drugs such as propranolol or oxprenolol, taken on a regular basis, are useful in lessening the frequency and severity of the pain and allowing the person to undertake more physical activity. Also, when angina is brought on by emotional stress rather than physical activity, beta blockers can be very effective.

They achieve their effect by a number of different mechanisms. In particular, they reduce the increase in heart rate which normally takes place in response to physical activity and emotion—the main precipitating causes of anginal pain. They also reduce the oxygen requirement of the heart muscle itself. But this type of therapy is not suitable for all: for instance, not for people with asthma or other diseases in which the airways are constricted, such as someone suffering from severe chronic bronchitis or from heart failure.

surgery for angina

If the quality of the person's life remains poor in spite of drug therapy (and there is no general contra-indication to an operation), further investigation may be undertaken to establish whether surgery would help. This requires investigation by coronary angiography in which a radio-opaque dye is injected into the coronary arteries so that they can be seen on cine X-ray. If this shows a localised obstruction in a major branch, it might be bypassed by what is known as coronary bypass grafting.

A short length (some 3 or 4 inches) is cut out from a vein in the leg. One end is placed above the obstruction, usually on the aorta, and the other below the obstruction in the coronary artery.

Following the operation, there is a very good chance that there will be no further anginal pain.

It would be difficult to prove that surgery prolongs the life of someone with angina. Although usually the quality of life improves a great deal, you must still be aware of factors which may have brought on the disease in the first place, such as smoking, overweight, stressful life-style—and avoid them.

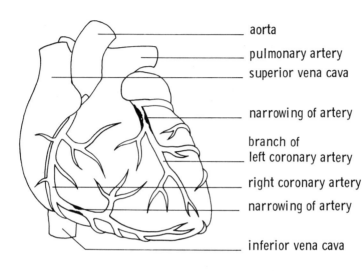

aorta

pulmonary artery

superior vena cava

narrowing of artery

branch of
left coronary artery

right coronary artery

narrowing of artery

inferior vena cava

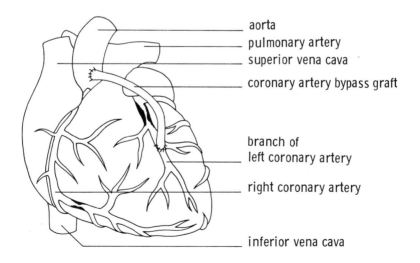

aorta

pulmonary artery

superior vena cava

coronary artery bypass graft

branch of
left coronary artery

right coronary artery

inferior vena cava

Coronary heart disease

The terms coronary heart disease, coronary artery disease, ischaemic heart disease refer to the process of narrowing of the coronary arteries which reduces the blood supply to the heart muscle. This is not synonymous with a heart attack but sets the stage for events such as angina and for myocardial infarction (also called cardiac infarct or coronary attack).

Myocardial infarction

When the narrowing of a branch of a coronary artery becomes so pronounced as to reduce the blood flow below a critical level, a blood clot may form (particularly if there is a temporary alteration in blood clotting power), and this clot then totally blocks up the artery. This is what is called a coronary thrombosis. The muscle beyond the obstruction which is dependent on that particular blood vessel for its supply, may then suffer. If collateral blood supply from another tributary vessel is sufficiently well developed, the event may pass unrecognised. Acute lack of blood to an area of the heart muscle can result in the death of that part of the heart muscle. This is what is known as a myocardial infarction.

It is most commonly due to a coronary thrombosis, but may also occur as a result of excessive demand on a heart with narrowed arteries. It may even occur without any obvious cause; this is the source of much current speculation and research. Possibilities include spasm of a coronary artery, disease of very small branches of the coronary arteries (too small to be visible by X-ray techniques, or at a post mortem), multiple tiny emboli, and disordered blood flow within the heart muscle.

Risk factors

Coronary heart disease accounts for approximately one third of all deaths in men over the age of 40 in Britain. Before the turn of the century it was relatively uncommon. It is possible that it was under-diagnosed in the past when modern investigative methods were not yet available. Also, many diseases that used to be fatal are now largely curable; this may have added to the impression of increase in recent years. Nevertheless, coronary heart disease is a common illness of our time and has been called the western way of death.

The phenomenal increase in coronary heart disease affects all age groups and both sexes and is particularly striking in younger men. The reason is far from clear; it has been put down to the modern affluent way of life, for want of something more precise. There is no apparent single cause but scientists have identified, by statistical appraisal, a number of factors which make a person more likely to develop the disease. Moreover, these risk factors all interact. The major ones which carry about equal amounts of risk are cigarette smoking, increased blood pressure and a high blood cholesterol. Other risk factors include heredity, the person's sex (men more prone than women) and personality, diabetes, a high level of triglycerides in the blood, and factors more in the control of the person, such as physical inactivity, stress, dietary factors, obesity, and oral contraceptives.

Different doctors put the various risk factors into slightly different orders of importance. There is genuine disagreement for instance about the relative importance of stress and fat. The controversy about the possible relationship between dietary fat and heart disease has not yet been resolved. The medical profession does not have—and does not claim to have—all the answers. The interaction of the various risk factors is probably more important than the relative significance of each of them alone.

A basic scientific principle is that the mere demonstration of a statistical correlation between a risk factor and a disease does not imply a cause-and-effect relationship. In other words, being able to show that, for example, raised blood pressure makes a person more liable to develop heart disease, does not imply that high blood pressure is the primary cause of heart disease or that the person will ever develop the disease. It is equally possible that another factor, factor x (for the sake of argument, stress) might cause raised blood pressure and, via other means, cause heart disease.

Cigarette smoking and coronary heart disease

Cigarette smoking is a self-imposed risk. Smoking 20 cigarettes a day approximately trebles the risk of dying from coronary disease before the age of 50. The risk of a non-fatal heart attack is also greater in cigarette smokers than non-smokers, particularly in younger men and women. However, within one year of giving up cigarette smoking, this extra risk is reduced to something between an eighth and a quarter.

The nicotine in cigarette smoke increases the amounts of adrenaline and noradrenaline released into the blood stream. This in turn has some effect on the release of lipids (cholesterol and triglycerides) into the blood stream. It is therefore possible that it increases the likelihood of atheroma forming. Even if cigarette smoking does not directly induce atheroma, it increases the effects of atheroma. Also, the release of adrenaline and noradrenaline into the blood stream increases the heart rate, and thus the work of the heart. It also increases the risk of ectopic beats.

The carbon monoxide content of cigarette smoke is remarkably high. Carbon monoxide combines with haemoglobin much more readily than oxygen, forming carboxyhaemoglobin. This dissociates only very slowly and is therefore competitive with oxygen, reducing the carrying power of the blood for oxygen. Inhaling deeply on one single cigarette can increase the level of carboxyhaemoglobin in the blood to about 15 per cent. This is particularly important in somebody whose coronary arteries are already narrowed so that the blood flow is restricted. If 15 per cent of the haemoglobin is not capable of transporting oxygen, this aggravates the effect of the lack of blood in the part of the heart beyond the narrowed artery.

Furthermore, the reduction of available oxygen in the coronary arteries is the very opposite of what is demanded by the increased heart rate brought about by the nicotine: having to work harder, the heart muscles need more oxygen—not less.

It is possible that the chronic carboxyhaemoglobinaemia increases the stickiness of the platelets, the components of the blood which play an important part in the process of blood coagulation: this in turn, may encourage the formation of clots within the vessels.

How to stop smoking

Giving up smoking is something you cannot do unless you really want to. Saying 'I suppose I ought to try and give it up' is not enough. You must feel really positive about it.

health and wealth
The first step is to think of all the reasons why you would be better off if you did not smoke. Some are only too obvious—for instance, if you have developed a smoker's cough or chronic bronchitis. When reading warnings that smoking can damage your health, lung cancer immediately springs to mind but the risk of a heart attack from cigarette smoking is even greater than the risk of lung cancer, which is the more feared. Changing to low tar cigarettes, or using filters,

may reduce the risk of lung cancer, but is thought unlikely to reduce that of coronary heart disease if the carbon monoxide yield is not also reduced. A pipe or cigar smoker probably incurs less risk, because generally he does not inhale. Switching from cigarette smoking to smoking either cigars or a pipe should reduce the risk but tends not to because cigarette smokers are used to inhaling and continue to inhale the smoke from the cigar or pipe.

Some people argue that they have known smokers who lived to a ripe old age, and are prepared to take a chance: 'You only die once', 'Each man to his poison'. It is true that people must be free to make their own choices but parents should reflect that smoking can damage their children's future—in more ways than one. The smoke from their cigarettes can turn their children into passive smokers. This is especially damaging to children under a year old. Moreover, it sets a bad example. The children of parents who smoke are more likely to smoke, too. It is an important consideration that by smoking in the home parents are encouraging their children to start smoking, waste money and damage their health. And a parent who smokes runs the risk of illness and premature death, possibly leaving behind a young family.

A pregnant woman should stop to ask herself whether it is fair to her unborn baby to make his choices for him. Each time she smokes, she passes nicotine and carbon monoxide through her bloodstream to the foetus. The newborn baby of a mother who smokes tends to be undersized and at a greater risk of retarded development than other babies. There is also a greater risk of miscarriage or stillbirth for a woman who continues smoking heavily after the fourth month of pregnancy.

Quite apart from damage to health, is the question of appearance.

Smoking a cigarette is no longer the symbol of cool sophistication that it used to be and, particularly in a heavy smoker, people are more likely to notice the unattractive debris in the ashtray, the stained fingers, and the pervasive smell of tobacco in the room, on your breath and clothes. The smoker may not be aware of this but it could well prove a turn-off for other people: a bad thing for the young and fancy-free—and even for the not so young.

You may find it helpful to make a list of your reasons for wanting to stop. It may help to increase your resolve later, particularly if some of the reasons are very personal ones.

Do not forget the cost: even for someone who has all the money he needs, it seems a pity to send it up in smoke.

Most important of all, do not be fatalistic about the whole thing. Many people imagine that if they have smoked for some time, the harm is done and there is no point in giving up. This is not true; it is never too late as far as giving up smoking is concerned. The increased risk of heart disease starts to fall immediately and continues to fall.

If you cannot stop altogether, cut down as much as possible—to five or less a day. Try not to inhale, and leave a one-third long stub.

strategy

Start planning your strategy by observing your own smoking habits. When do you smoke? Why do you smoke? What do you get out of it?

It could be useful to fill in a 24-hour smoking chart. Every time you reach for a cigarette, make a note of the time and what you were doing at the time: reading, drinking coffee, taking a break, getting down to a piece of work, watching TV, meeting acquaintances in a pub, having a frustrating phone call or a difficult interview. Record your mood at the time and your reason for smoking that particular cigarette, if you know it. Are you, for instance, rewarding yourself for some unpleasant job you have just done, or is it simply habit and you hardly know you are doing it?

Different people smoke for different reasons, and a person can smoke for different reasons at different times. Amongst the main reasons are stimulation, reduction of tension, pleasure, habit, ritual. Try to discover which of these apply to you.

for stimulation
Stimulation smokers use cigarettes to wake themselves up and to keep going. If this applies to you, you could try taking a brisk walk or moderate exercise instead, breathing slowly and deeply or taking a mildly stimulating drink such as tea or coffee.

reduce tension
If you smoke to reduce tension, try to divert your tension by some activity: chewing gum or liquorice, sucking a mint, eating fruit or nibbling (a low-calorie food); also—depending on where you happen to be at the time—splashing cold water on your face, neck and arms; practising relaxation (yoga or keep-fit classes could help), breathing deeply.

All smokers who are trying to stop should teach themselves a simple form of relaxation to use when they feel tense, or badly in want of a cigarette. One method is to sit (or preferably lie) in a comfortable position, then tense the muscles of the feet and let go, then the muscles of the legs and let go, next the thighs and so on, travelling up the body until all muscles have been tensed and then relaxed in turn. You should then make sure that you feel relaxed all over, and if you find that, for instance, the muscles in your shoulders are taut, hunch them up and then let them go. Do not forget the face muscles— mouth, eyes and brow should feel soft and relaxed.

mainly for pleasure?
If you smoke mainly for pleasure, you will need to find some alternative source of satisfaction. Change your pattern of activity, particularly after meals and in tea (or coffee) breaks.

Pleasure from smoking can turn into a craving for tobacco. This can reach the point where putting out one cigarette triggers off the desire for another one. If you are in this situation, you cannot hope to give up gradually—nothing short of a clean break will work. The first week will be very tough but the second will not be as continuously bad. You must accept bouts of craving and be prepared for possible withdrawal symptoms. In the first few days, there may be some nausea, pallor, shakiness, irritability and some difficulty in sleeping and concentrating. The nausea usually passes very quickly, the other symptoms can continue for some time. The craving may also return at intervals.

There is no drug that consistently helps withdrawal. A smoker who feels the need to put something into his mouth could try a dummy cigarette. There are lozenges and chewing gum which make cigarettes taste awful, and filters to put into a cigarette holder, designed to remove some of the tar and nicotine, to help break the smoker's dependence.

Some addicts have stopped smoking by developing an aversion to it through chain smoking non-stop for two days, or until they could not bear the thought of another cigarette—and then stopping, never to smoke again. But this can be a dangerous method: do not try it without consulting your doctor first.

kick the habit
If you are a habit smoker and light up frequently without realising it, you must first of all become more conscious of what you are doing. There are some tricks you can try to break your habit patterns. Ask yourself each time 'Do I really need this cigarette? what satisfaction will it give me?' Then try doing everything differently so that it is no longer automatic: carry your cigarettes in a different pocket, wrap them up in paper and a rubber band, try lighting up with the other hand, do not carry a lighter or matches. If you always reach for a cigarette when you telephone, pick up the receiver with the other hand—the hand you would use for holding the cigarette; if you do not know how the cigarette in your mouth got there, stub it out. Other ploys are to be out of stock by never buying a fresh pack until the old pack is empty. Try keeping your cigarettes in an inaccessible spot—on a high shelf, in a drawer or in a room in which you do not normally smoke. Give them to someone else so that you have to ask for each cigarette.

If your daily routine would seem very odd without cigarettes, change your routine and so break your conditioned reflexes. Try varying the time and place of your activities. Avoid situations where other people are smoking. See if you can arrange to work in the company of non-smokers.

ritual
Some people, far from being unaware of their smoking habits, derive their main pleasure from the ritual that accompanies each cigarette.

They enjoy the handling itself. Handlers enjoy opening a crisp new pack, going through the motions of taking out a cigarette, tapping it, striking the match, lighting the cigarette, being conscious of handling it and watching the smoke. Instead, you might toy with a pencil, doodle, play with a coin, an executive toy, a piece of jewellery, or worry beads.

the tempters
It might be a good idea to tell people that you are giving up: this can help your resolve, so as not to lose face by weakening. On the other hand, secrecy may be more helpful: let your colleagues notice your abstinence first.

Decide how you are going to deal with your smoking friends if they try to tempt you—some people take a perverse pleasure in causing the fall of a reformed smoker. On the other hand, you may find your spouse or a friend prepared to try and give up with you. Or you could enquire from your local health authority whether there is a smoking withdrawal group in your area. If not, you could perhaps form an informal one with your friends.

stop!

Be sure to choose a good day on which to start the campaign—not when you are under stress. This could be when you go away on holiday or at the start of a weekend, but if you tend to smoke more when you are relaxing and enjoying yourself, stop on a monday morning! If you have 'flu or some other illness during which you are unable to smoke, do not go back to it afterwards. This applies all the more if you have had a heart attack.

The biggest decision to make is whether to stop outright or cut down gradually until you stop altogether. The best thing is to stop at once.

But if you cannot altogether do that, you should at least set yourself a date for starting the cut back and a time limit of, say, no more than a month, at the end of which you will have cut down your smoking to zero.

Generally, the most successful quitters stop suddenly after a period of preparation. If it seems an impossible hardship to think that you will never smoke another cigarette, take things one day at a time and say to yourself 'I will not have a cigarette today'. Encourage yourself by using the money you are saving by not smoking to buy yourself something specific that you would otherwise do without. Work out what three months' smoking costs you now and, if you have the cash, go out and spend it in anticipation of your success—on new clothes, a weekend away or perhaps even a holiday. If you buy something tangible, each time you use it (or wear it or look at it) it will remind you that you now possess it because you no longer smoke.

Having chosen a propitious day on which to stop, make sure the evening before that you have no cigarettes left—destroying the remaining ones is a useful and symbolic action.

Stopping smoking often brings about a conflict of interests in that many people put on weight. However, obesity, for all its attendant problems, is by far the lesser of the two evils as far as coronary heart disease is concerned.

If you find that you put on weight when you stop, this could be because your sense of taste improves and so you enjoy your food more and therefore eat more. Or maybe you use food to fill the gap left by tobacco. This should right itself after a time, particularly if you are careful to avoid high Calorie foods (anything fatty or sweet); and to take more exercise. Ex-smokers on the whole end up by gaining not more than 2 to 3 pounds on average, although they tend to put on a lot more to begin with.

This does not mean that people should be complacent about getting fat. But it is usually a bad plan to attempt to stop smoking and reduce weight at the same time. If giving up smoking results in an increase in weight, this can be dealt with at a later stage.

publications
In the interest of national health, much detailed advice and information has been published to help smokers to stop or at least cut down. Publications include:

The smoker's guide to non-smoking, a booklet published by the Health Education Council as part of their *Look After Yourself* campaign;

written by a clinical psychologist, complete with a plan of action including charts for you to fill in (your reasons for stopping, daily records, smoking situations and even a ready reckoner so that you can work out how much you are saving);

available from the Health Education Council, 78 New Oxford Street, London WC1A 1AH, tel: 01-637 1881.

Reports Action, published by ASH (Action on Smoking and Health)

looks like a daily newspaper and contains good articles on why do you smoke, 21 steps to help you quit, devising a plan, doing it gradually, what to expect;

available from ASH, 27–35 Mortimer Street, London W1N 7RJ, tel: 01-637 9843.

How to stop smoking, a leaflet produced by the Scottish Health

Education Group, Woodburn House, Canaan Lane, Edinburgh. The Ulster Cancer Foundation, 40 Eglantine Avenue, Belfast, also produces some relevant anti-smoking publications.

A report on smoking was published in *Which?* August 1980. It looks at the prevalence and risks of smoking, and examines methods which smokers can try to help them give up, for example clinics, manuals and acupuncture. The general conclusion is that nothing replaces the need for will-power, and no one method is markedly more successful than another. The report also describes measures, such as increased taxation and advertising restrictions, which attempt to reduce smoking on a national scale.

Raised blood pressure

The concept is no longer held that there is such a thing as a normal blood pressure, with a definite threshold above which blood pressure should be considered as 'high'. There is a sliding scale of pressure from low to high with no cut-off points; the risk increases all along the line. In other words, within reason, the lower the pressure the better, and the higher, the worse—particularly in an older person.

Raised blood pressure incurs approximately the same order of risk of coronary heart disease as cigarette smoking. With cigarette smoking, the risk decreases rapidly when the habit is discontinued. There is as yet no firm evidence that treating high blood pressure improves the outlook as far as a heart attack is concerned. Lowering raised blood pressure is a definite factor in reducing the risk of stroke and the early results of studies now in progress encourage the belief that such treatment also helps to decrease the death rate from coronary heart disease.

Even though the theory that reducing the risk of coronary heart disease by treating raised blood pressure is at the moment still unproven, it is better to take the benefit of the doubt and seek treatment. Doctors recommend that people of any age should have their blood pressure checked at least once every two years. The next time you see your general practitioner, for whatever reason, ask him if he will measure your blood pressure.

What can go wrong as a result of raised blood pressure

There do not seem to be any very specific symptoms ascribable to raised blood pressure itself, except in the most extreme cases of gross hypertension. It is a commonly held belief that symptoms such as headache, dizziness, palpitations, fatigue and lack of concentration may be symptoms of hypertension. Such symptoms often lead the person to visit his doctor and during the course of the examination hypertension may or may not be found.

There is no apparent single cause of raised blood pressure. Although some kidney disease can cause hypertension and severe hypertension can lead to kidney damage, they are not inevitably cause and effect. In one or two types of raised blood pressure where the cause is known (such as glandular disorder, or malformation or inflammation of the kidneys, or toxaemia of pregnancy) it can usually be corrected. But most types of hypertension fall into the group known as essential hypertension, a singularly unhappy description since the last thing it is is 'essential' in the colloquial sense. Medically, the term means that doctors do not know the cause.

Amongst the likely risks of raised blood pressure are heart failure and stroke.

hypertensive heart failure

Raised blood pressure can result in a thickening of the left ventricular muscle and this can ultimately lead to left heart failure. This hypertensive heart failure, when the thickened heart muscle eventually outgrows its own blood supply, is usually manifest by undue breathlessness on exertion, difficulty in breathing when lying down, sometimes acute attacks of breathlessness particularly in the middle of the night. If left untreated, it could be followed by failure of the right side of the heart. This is associated with an increase of fluid volume in the body, manifest by swelling of the legs and sometimes distension of the abdomen or swelling of the liver.

stroke

Another major complication of high blood pressure is the risk of a stroke.

The word stroke is sometimes rather loosely used to describe a heart attack. This is wrong. The word stroke should be confined to damage to the brain which is caused when a blood vessel in the brain either bursts (haemorrhage) or is blocked by a blood clot, and the consequences of this.

A stroke caused by haemorrhage is easy to understand if we return to the parallel with the central heating system. Imagine what it would be like if the pressure was doubled in the hot water circuit: something would have to give. What usually gives is one of the small arteries within the brain, particularly if there happens to be a slight inherent weakness in any one part of the wall of the artery.

Hypertension is associated with increased atherosclerosis (the furring up of arteries through the deposit of atheroma) in the lining of the arteries. Eventually the narrowing of the arteries may reach a critical point so that the blood flow is slowed up. This encourages the formation of clots, which may subsequently block the blood vessel, or be dislodged and carried in the blood stream to form a blockage in one of the smaller arteries which are too narrow to let it pass. (This is called an embolism.) A clot in an artery of the brain blocks off the blood supply to part of brain, causes damage to that part, and may be fatal. If the person survives, he is usually affected or even paralysed in those parts of the body controlled by the particular part of the brain that has been damaged.

Treatment of raised blood pressure

It would seem reasonable to try and reduce excess stress, because emotional stress is quite capable of raising the blood pressure. Excessive increase in physical exertion is probably best avoided.

The doctor will advise on diet. There is disagreement about the effect of salt in the diet. Some doctors have noted a dramatic effect on some patients who have been made to adhere to a low-salt diet; others consider it unproven. At present, there is no hard evidence that less salt in the nation's diet would widely lower blood pressure levels.

Anyone who is overweight will be firmly told by his doctor to reduce weight. This may be enough to control borderline or mildly raised blood pressure. Also, hypotensive drugs (drugs to lower blood pressure) tend to be relatively ineffective in an overweight person, particularly someone grossly obese.

drugs
Many physicians are of the opinion that anyone with diastolic pressures of between 95 and 110 mmHg should be treated if there are other associated risk factors, such as a history of cigarette smoking or diabetes. And people with a diastolic pressure of over 115 to 120 mmHg are likely to be given treatment to help protect them from most of the complications.

The complications of hypertension such as stroke and heart failure can only be avoided if the blood pressure is continuously controlled. This will mean regular attendance at the surgery to assess progress and maintain medication. Much will depend on the enthusiasm of the person to be treated and his determination to take tablets regularly.

High blood pressure tends to be a fluctuating problem, requiring regular supervision: as the level of blood pressure goes up and down owing to environmental factors and other (unknown) factors, so the dose of medication may need adjusting.

The hypotensive drugs used to have many unpleasant side effects, so that the treatment was considered worse than the disease. In recent years, the medication has improved enormously.

First, the person is generally given diuretics, maybe combined with a potassium supplement to replace the excessive potassium loss that the diuretics bring about. The diuretics may, if necessary, be supplemented with a beta-blocking agent. The precise mechanisms involved in both these lines of treatment are not fully understood. If necessary, stronger medication may be added or substituted, such as potent vasodilators, or drugs that act by an effect within the central nervous system.

side effects
Each powerful agent can produce particular side effects. If your doctor does not warn you, ask him what kinds of side effects you might expect.

Generally, the stronger medications have greater incidence of side effects such as impotence, fainting and postural hypotension. This is a feeling of faintness when standing up quickly, particularly when standing up out of a hot bath. Hypotensive drugs increase this effect because, as part of the treatment, they prevent the increase in blood pressure that is necessary in normal circumstances. We are physiologically adapted to increase our blood pressure very quickly so that when we stand up suddenly the pressure increases: it is this which is counteracted by some of these drugs, and can be associated with fainting. The habit has to be learned of always rising slowly from the lying or sitting position. Somebody who is particularly sensitive to postural hypotension and is given hypotensive drugs should tell his doctor because he might be better off with different drugs.

In some elderly people, the side effects may outweigh the benefits of the hypotensive drug and the doctor may decide, on balance, not to prescribe any.

do-it-yourself monitoring

In the USA, there are pay machines in some shops and pharmacies at which people can take their own blood pressure readings. In this country, do-it-yourself sphygmomanometers are offered for sale to the public. While having your blood pressure checked by a doctor every so often is a good thing, it would be exaggerated to recommend that people should buy a self-determination blood pressure measurer.

There are, however, a few instances when taking your own blood pressure may be recommended by the doctor. A patient on long-term medication for high blood pressure, particularly someone whose condition is deteriorating, can avoid having to make frequent clinic visits by taking his own blood pressure readings. He then needs to attend at the clinic only when there has been a significant change in his blood pressure, so that his dosage may be adjusted.

By taking their own measurements, people with widely fluctuating blood pressure can be helped to recognise events which raise their blood pressure, such as various types of stress, and then avoid these situations.

Most people can be taught how to take their own blood pressure if the doctor wishes them to do so. (The basic equipment is similar to what the doctor uses, with a dial instead of a column of mercury. The cuff of the sphygmomanometer is fastened with velcro and can therefore be fastened with one hand. The readings are indicated by flashes or bleeps.)

The proposed introduction of coin-in-the-slot blood pressure testing machines in sports centres and other public places is not being welcomed by the medical profession.

Cholesterol, and fats

Cholesterol is a complex fat-like substance which is essential to the body, as part of cell membranes and for the making of steroid hormones and male and female sex hormones. Cholesterol is carried around the body by the blood stream, in which it is one of the plasma lipids.

Cholesterol is the main component of the fatty deposits in the lining of the arteries (atheroma). Experimental evidence derived from animals which have been fed on mainly cholesterol-containing foods showed that they developed fatty deposits in the arteries similar to, but probably not identical with, atheroma.

Various studies have shown a positive relationship between levels of blood cholesterol in a community and the occurrence of coronary heart disease. In individual people, too, it seems that the blood cholesterol level can give an indication of the likelihood of coronary heart disease: the higher the level, the greater the risk.

The fact that high blood cholesterol levels are statistically associated with an increased risk of heart disease does not necessarily imply a cause-and-effect relationship.

The risk of an individual with high blood cholesterol developing coronary heart disease is greater if the person also has raised blood pressure or diabetes or smokes cigarettes.

At present, there is conflicting evidence about reducing the risk of coronary heart disease by lowering a raised cholesterol level. Methods of lowering cholesterol are only partially effective. This may be because dietary changes are not radical enough, or drug treatment may not be given in high enough doses because of toxicity problems.

To prevent coronary heart disease may require that the cholesterol is lowered substantially; the treatment may need to be prolonged or started early enough in life to prevent rather than get rid of atheroma.

diet and cholesterol

Most of the body's supply of cholesterol is made by the body in the liver and other organs; the rest comes from certain foods in the diet. This dietary cholesterol is found mainly in egg yolk, butter, liver and kidney.

But it seems that it is not so much the amount of dietary cholesterol that affects the cholesterol concentration in the blood stream as the amount and type of fat a person eats. Fat includes butter, margarine and lard, also cooking oil (liquid fat) and fat on meat; there is also non-visible fat in most other foods. Many kinds of cheese contain nearly 40 per cent fat, and chocolate does, too.

Fats are composed of a mixture of fatty acids. There are several dozen fatty acids in nature, which accounts for the variety and individual character of natural fats. Fatty acids are made up, chemically, of carbon, hydrogen and oxygen and their individual properties depend on the length of the carbon chain and the extent to which it can combine with hydrogen atoms. A fatty acid is said to be saturated when the carbon chain contains as many hydrogen atoms as it can hold; in mono-unsaturated fatty acids there are two hydrogen atoms missing in the carbon chain. If four or more hydrogen atoms are missing in a chain, the fatty acid is said to be polyunsaturated.

Fat-containing foods in our diet consist of a mixture of fatty acids and no food is purely saturated or purely unsaturated. However, most can be classified as predominantly saturated, or predominantly mono-unsaturated or predominantly polyunsaturated.

Saturated fatty acids are found mainly in the solid fats of animal origin, such as those in butter and meat; also some plant products such as coconut. Most vegetable fatty acids are predominantly unsaturated and, as such, are liquid or soft at room temperatures. When liquid oils are hardened as in the manufacture of margarine, unsaturated fatty acids are changed into saturated fatty acids.

Saturated fatty acids in the diet increase the blood cholesterol concentration, while polyunsaturated fats in the diet tend to lower it. Some studies have suggested that the saturated fat content of the diet is the single most important factor in raising blood cholesterol levels and that this is associated with the development of coronary heart disease. However, blood fat levels are also influenced by individual rates of fat metabolism in the body and by genetic factors.

recommended diet?
It is not possible to make categoric recommendations about foods to eat and foods to avoid. Many doctors consider it prudent to advise people to limit their overall fat intake in order to lower blood cholesterol, in the hope that this will give a measure of protection against coronary heart disease. They suggest cutting down particularly on foods high in saturated fats (fats of animal origin or hardened fat) and partly replacing them by foods high in polyunsaturated fats.

Foods to go easy on would therefore include eggs (because of their high cholesterol content), butter, cream, lard, suet, hard margarine and 'soft' margarine containing hardened fat, coconut oil, chocolate, meat fat, and meat generally. Fish and poultry are preferable to meat because they contain a lower proportion of saturated fat and are a good source of polyunsaturated fatty acids.

Grilling is a better method than frying and any cooking oils used should be high in polyunsaturated fats, for instance corn oil, or sunflower oil. Oils that are simply called 'vegetable oil' should preferably not be used as they may contain a high proportion of saturated fat.

Cakes and pastries also contain fats and eating somewhat less of them can result in a worthwhile reduction in fat in the diet.

Vegetables and fruit should figure prominently in everyone's diet.

This pattern of eating is also good for anyone who wants to lose weight or to maintain their weight at a sensible level.

Triglycerides

Triglycerides are also blood fats which, in excess, may predispose the person towards coronary disease. The risk associated with a raised level of triglycerides is not as high as that of cholesterol. The substance which narrows the coronary arteries, atheroma, is composed approximately of 2/3rds cholesterol and 1/3rd triglycerides. Too great a consumption of alcohol can increase triglyceride levels in some people; it is also thought that the levels tend to be raised by a high intake of carbohydrates, particularly sugar, and animal fats.

Stress

Not all doctors place the same significance on emotional stress as a factor in the development of heart attacks; the effects of emotional stress are not all measurable and are therefore difficult to quantify.

However, some studies have been carried out in which heart beat, blood pressure and other physiological responses were monitored in conditions of stress, in both normal subjects and people with coronary disease. They showed that emotion can be powerful in influencing the heart rate, comparable to the most intense physical exercise.

The ostensibly mild and everyday emotional stress of driving a car in busy town traffic along a known route has been shown to produce a maximum heart rate between 100 and 140 beats per minute (averaging approximately 110, compared with resting levels of about 60 to 80 beats per minute). To bring about this degree of speeding up the heart's action by physical activity, an amount of exercise roughly equivalent to walking at a brisk pace or climbing a flight of stairs would be required.

The more intense emotional challenge of speaking before an audience has been shown to produce heart rates of between about 120 and 170 beats per minute (averaging, in one study, about 150). More often than not, the person is unaware of the increased rate.

The severe emotional challenges of anticipating a first descent from an aeroplane by parachute, and of racing car driving, have both been shown to produce heart rates consistently above 180 beats per minute, reaching as much as 200 beats per minute. This would compare with maximum physical exertion. Yet, in the case of the parachutists, they were sitting absolutely still anticipating the event, hardly moving a muscle. Similarly, the amount of movement actually possible within the confines of a racing car is virtually limited to toe raising, gear changing and small movements of the steering wheel.

In the studies, the electrocardiogram was monitored. The wave form pattern in subjects with normal hearts changed under stress (such as parachute jumping) in a manner comparable to the way it changes with exercise in people with coronary disease.

stress causing atheroma

A hypothesis has been advanced to explain why prolonged stress may influence the development of atheroma. Under conditions of stress, increased amounts of the sympathetic hormones adrenaline and nor-adrenaline are released, the concentrations very roughly parallelling the degree of stress. This increase results in the liberation of free fatty acids into the blood stream (to provide a source of energy). However, in the absence of physical exercise, this fat is not burned up; it becomes converted by the liver into triglyceride and, to a lesser extent, into cholesterol which become available to be incorporated into atheroma deposits. (Perhaps human bodies are environmentally better adapted for a primitive type of existence where emotional challenge is automatically associated with some form of physical action or combat.)

Apart from the short-term studies of various stress situations which support this theory, there was a longer term study of two groups of accountants. One group was made up of tax accountants whose deadlines occurred in April, the other company accountants whose deadlines occurred in January. Both groups showed a rise in blood cholesterol prior to the balance-sheet time of year.

falling heart rate

Not all emotional stress situations are associated with an increased heart rate. Anticipating, witnessing, or actually experiencing pain can cause a reduction in heart rate. Having dental treatment is one example when the heart rate may actually fall, before the dentist even touches you (in other words, in anticipation of possible pain), and rise again to the original values after the dentist has finished.

One of the people who was monitored with a portable electrocardiograph when jumping from an aeroplane by parachute, fractured his leg on landing. There was a delay of about 2 minutes before he experienced pain. The heart rate fell sharply from about 185 to 55 beats per minute immediately he hit the ground. This was despite extremely high adrenaline concentrations circulating in the blood. The parasympathetic nervous system, which has the opposite effect to the sympathetic system (ie slows the heart rate) completely overrode the sympathetic system. The same applied in the situations of anticipating dental treatment, and while watching violence on film. In both these situations, the parasympathetic nervous system dominated although greatly increased activity of the sympathetic system was shown by analysis of urine and blood samples.

In the film-watching studies, the heart rate fell appreciably during the scenes of violence, but the people watching were under the impression that, if anything, they had a fast heart rate. They described their heart as pounding in the chest or throbbing in the throat. In fact, this is a common fallacy, since an awareness of this throbbing or pounding is associated with increased force of contraction which in turn is associated with increased filling of the heart and an increased volume of blood that is ejected.

Stress, and personality

While not all doctors agree that prolonged emotional stress will by itself lead to heart trouble, it is likely to be important in a person with other risk factors, such as a cigarette smoker or one with raised blood pressure. This is particularly so in a workaholic, self-driving, time-conscious, aggressive type of person.

The effects of emotional stress can creep up on a person in an insidious manner, so that he is hardly aware of the extent to which this has occurred. An example is what cardiologists have described as the pre-coronary syndrome in a middle-aged man climbing the ladder of his profession with all the energy and tenacity of an active, competitive man. For a variety of reasons, possibly lack of holiday and domestic or work pressures, he becomes conscious of lagging behind a little and equally conscious of the hot breath of his junior competitors coming up behind him. He combats this by working even harder; taking work home in the evening, after staying late at the office. As a result, he gets more tired and his work, if anything, tends to slow down still more. He is now taking work home at the weekends as well. Such recreational activities as he may have previously indulged in have long gone by the board, because he has 'absolutely no time to spare'. Any thought of taking a holiday is now totally out of the question. A vicious circle is set up and such a person is a likely victim of a heart attack.

If this spiral of events is pointed out to him, he may resist any suggestion that he break the vicious circle, or force himself to take time off. 'I cannot afford 4 hours a week for sport and relaxation, I cannot afford 4 minutes'. People who say that it is just not possible to delegate in their particular work should face up to the fact that if they do not do so voluntarily, they may end up taking an enforced rest in the intensive care unit of a hospital.

People who realise the situation in time and do something about it, even if it is no more than taking regular holidays, can become transformed. Returning refreshed and relaxed, the pile of seemingly insuperable problems and difficulties which has been amassing is often swept aside or overcome in no time at all.

There can be few more fatuous phrases in the english language than 'try not to worry'. Very few people have the ability consciously to dismiss a monumental worry from their mind. This is where exercise is of use, since it is difficult for most of us to worry about disagreeable prospects and personal, financial, or work problems when chasing a ball across a court or indulging in some form of fairly fast moving physical activity. Although it is difficult to prove this, exercise is probably one of the most effective anti-stress measures available.

Yoga may make a person feel more at ease and relaxed and can therefore be of some benefit.

Yoga teachers call it a way of life that people practice in order to find new avenues of spiritual and physical development. The postures and the breathing techniques systematically exercise the whole body and are said to improve the circulation of the blood throughout the body. The aim of the discipline is that the mind, too, should become clearer so that everyday tensions of life will dissolve.

Even without the formal discipline of yoga, it is useful to learn a few relaxation exercises such as alternating a tensing and a flopping activity, for instance hunching the shoulders up towards the ears, tensing the muscles—and then dropping the shoulders and relaxing. All the parts of the body can be worked and then relaxed in such a way. Regular short sessions of such clench-and-let-go exercises can be a useful antidote to stress.

Physical inactivity

There is some evidence that physical inactivity plays a part in the development of coronary heart disease—although this has been particularly difficult to evaluate. One study, for example, showed a lesser incidence of death from heart attack in conductors of double-decker buses in London than in drivers, and also a greater incidence in government clerks than in postmen. However, any simple cause-and-effect relationship was challenged by the observation that the bus drivers were fatter than the conductors and therefore may have been of a different metabolic type. It is also possible that people may become drivers because other factors, such as smoking habits and personality, make them appreciate a sedentary occupation more.

The main problem in many studies associating sedentary occupations with an increased incidence of coronary heart disease is that the persons concerned may pre-select themselves without realising it. In other words, someone who decides to be a bus driver, sitting down, with its minimal physical effort (as against a conductor running up and down stairs) may do so because he dislikes physical exercise. It is difficult to disentangle the other variables from the question of physical activity.

The same may apply to the person who pursues some form of sport throughout most of his life, as against a person who does his best to avoid it. The latter may do so because he smokes too much or overworks and, again, these other factors may be more important than the exercise or lack of it.

While none of the studies have shown that prolonged physical inactivity leads to coronary heart disease, a study of middle-aged sedentary employees has shown the protective nature of physical activity. The incidence of coronary heart disease amongst those whose activities included vigorous pursuits such as swimming, running, cycling, climbing many stairs, active gardening, was about one third of those who did not.

the value of exercise

Contrary to popular belief, such evidence as there is about exercise protecting against coronary heart disease is controversial.

Whatever exercise does or does not do in terms of preventing coronary heart disease, at least it makes the person feel better, look better, work better, perform almost all bodily functions better (including improving sex, and helping to combat obesity). So it is not to be discouraged—quite the opposite.

However, before rushing out and buying a tracksuit and joining the fashionable set, consider carefully what sort of exercise to undertake. Young, healthy people (say, under about thirty) should be encouraged to undertake anything they wish, with all the vigour and enthusiasm at their command. As the years advance, however, even the apparently healthy should apply a little caution and forego the more energetic and aggressive sports. This particularly applies to people who have abandoned sport, perhaps in their 20s, and then one day at the age of 45, glancing in the mirror and disliking what they see, resolve to rectify the situation in the shortest possible time. This is a potentially hazardous situation, particularly if the person has abandoned sport in the first place in order to devote all his energy and time to his work. If he then applies the same tenacity and determination to the process of getting fit and making up the 20 years' inactivity in the space of 45 minutes on a squash court, he is likely to do himself far more harm than good.

The tired, middle-aged, overworked and flabby should bear in mind a set of rules:

○ Do not take undue exercise when you are not feeling well, or recovering from influenza or a bad cold. Many men think they can 'work it off' and may do themselves harm. (If you are not sure, check first with your doctor.)

○ If possible, exercise should be enjoyable or at least not distasteful.

○ Start with only short periods of exercise, and gradually and regularly work up through a period of weeks.

○ Never ignore fatigue, always take a rest when tired.

○ Avoid exercising to the point of pain, severe breathlessness or distress.

○ Avoid isometric exercises, that is, the application of great force to a heavy load (as in weight-lifting) or to some immovable object. Press-ups are probably the most common example of this: although the arms are moving, most of the effort is contained in keeping the trunk rigid without movement. Isometric exercise raises the blood pressure enormously and may therefore be dangerous for someone predisposed to heart disease. Isotonic or dynamic exercises are infinitely preferable; the best examples are swimming, during which the arms and legs are constantly on the move, also walking, cycling, tennis, badminton, dancing.

For most people, time is a factor and this together with the lack of available sports facilities probably largely accounts for the spread of jogging. Jogging is something between walking and running; it does not make tremendous demands on the body and can be done at various speeds. It is best to start by jogging a short distance then walking and then jogging again, increasing the jogging and decreasing the walking stretches progressively. It depends on the person's fitness for how long he should sustain jogging.

However, if jogging or any other sport or exercise brings on pain in the chest, make sure you consult your doctor.

Men, women and heredity

Men are more prone to developing coronary heart disease than women. It is speculated that women may be hormonally protected until the time of the menopause. After that, the predominance of male heart attacks relative to women's decreases, until at about the age of 70-plus the two become similar.

But there has been an increase of heart disease in younger women since about 1960. It could be that young women are smoking more these days, and that the relative increase of smoking in young women in the war years may have started to show its effect 20 years later, or possibly because women are taking a more masculine role in society in terms of work commitments and the extra stresses that this involves. The effect of taking oral contraceptives in women over 35 may also be a factor.

medical check-up

A bad family history, namely close relatives who have suffered from coronary heart disease, high blood pressure, diabetes, or had a stroke, or who died comparatively young (that is, below about the age of 60) would indicate an increased risk. But unless several members of the family are involved, the risk is less than from the three factors of smoking, high blood pressure and high cholesterol level.

People in this group would be well advised to be aware of, and not to increase, their own risk. While routinely screening the whole population would be extravagant and probably non-productive, a person whose parents or siblings pointed to the risk, should get regular and thorough check-ups. For instance, an inherited fatty disorder of the blood can be modified by diet and the help of drugs and so the risk reduced.

People sometimes ask their general practitioner for a check-up because they want to make sure that no damage has so far been done and if everything appears to be all right, are inclined to take this as a sign that they can carry on safely as they are, without worrying about smoking or stress or exercise.

Having a check-up is not enough unless the people in whom any risk factors are discovered or confirmed are willing to adjust their life-style, including not smoking and watching their diet.

diabetes

A person at risk from diabetes may be identified through a routine examination. There is a higher incidence of heart trouble amongst people suffering from diabetes than in non-diabetics. Also, atherosclerosis is more common.

It has not been shown conclusively that early and effective treatment of diabetes reduces the incidence of the effects on blood vessels, but it seems reasonable to accept that this is so. In any case, early detection of diabetes is inevitably good for the control of that disease.

Diabetes is often associated with obesity, high blood fat levels and sometimes raised blood pressure, and much of the increased risk from diabetes is probably due to the interaction of these factors.

Obesity and dietary factors

It used to be widely held that being overweight carried considerably increased risk of developing heart disease. Recently, more sophisticated appraisal of available data has shown that the risk of coronary heart disease is significantly increased only if there are other risk factors, particularly diabetes or raised blood pressure and a raised level of cholesterol or triglycerides in the blood.

Nevertheless, it is a fact that obesity makes a person more liable to suffer from diabetes and raised blood pressure, and the association of these factors increases the risk of coronary heart disease.

Losing weight is a good thing even if it does not directly lower the risk of coronary heart disease. It is recommended as tending to reduce fat concentration in the blood, particularly triglycerides, and reducing raised blood pressure, and having a beneficial effect in diabetes.

losing weight

When trying to lose weight, it is better to think in terms of achieving a sensible eating pattern which you can follow permanently, rather than a 'diet'.

The way to lose weight is by eating less or eating differently, to reduce the overall number of Calories you take in. When your intake of Calories (your energy intake) is lower than your energy expenditure, your body will draw on its stores of fat to make up the deficit, and you therefore lose weight. Using up more energy by being more active also helps. An energy gap of 3500 Calories breaks down 1 lb of fat in the body.

The average number of Calories required by a moderately active normally-built man is about 2750 to 2900 a day, depending on age, and for a moderately active woman, it is about 2150. Slimming usually involves reducing one's total daily intake so as to create an energy gap of about 1000 Calories. In one week it should be possible to lose about 2 lbs by taking in 1000 Calories less than the normal requirement each day. To do this, it is worth becoming familiar with the calorific value of the foodstuffs you eat, so as to be able to calculate what your daily intake was before you started slimming, and to adjust it in order to slim. The various slimming methods are described in detail in the book *Which? way to slim.*

While the calorific content of the diet should be reduced, it is important to remember that you need a certain amount of protein every day and should have a healthy balanced diet with plenty of fresh fruit and vegetables, and not too much fat. Fats are particularly high in Calories, quite apart from possibly being a contributory factor to coronary heart disease. So you should try to reduce your intake of fats: the body needs only very small amounts of fat.

The main sources of carbohydrates in the diet are bread, flour, cereals, sugar, potatoes; except for sugar, they all contain other nutrients useful for the body. Sugar has no nutritional value other than its energy content.

There is no clear evidence in the available information to show that ordinary intake of sugar is, by itself, a risk factor in coronary heart disease. The assertion has been made in the past that high consumption of sugar is associated with increased risk of coronary heart disease. But there is no firm evidence for this either. However, in some people, a high sugar intake can raise blood triglyceride levels, and a high sugar consumption can lead to obesity which in turn is often associated with other risk factors. And, in all events, cutting down on sugar consumption is certainly an important factor in slimming. So, go easy on cakes, pastries, puddings, biscuits, sweets.

Dietary fibre, the fibrous structure of cereals, vegetables and fruit which cannot be digested by the body, does not supply energy. The effect of fibre in the diet in preventing coronary heart disease is at present no more than speculative. It is certain, however, that it is useful in preventing constipation.

crash diet?
Weight loss should be gradual and progressive. Whatever energy gap you set, you will lose more weight in the first week of slimming than later because in the first week you lose several pounds of water as well as fat. The only advantage of a fairly severe dietary programme for a couple of weeks, during which half a stone or even more may be lost, is the psychological boost of watching the pounds melt away. This may help in encouraging the person to go on with a more gradual, long-term scheme. But any drastic 'crash' slimming should not be attempted for any length of time (two weeks at most), and the diet should be suggested by a doctor.

Alcohol

There is no evidence that modest amounts of alcohol, such as a glass of sherry, a single whisky or a pint or two of beer do any damage to a healthy heart. Large or frequent amounts, however, can do progressive harm.

Alcohol is of high calorific value and should be avoided when slimming. Not only does alcohol in quantity taken daily or frequently lead to obesity, but also to an increased amount of blood fats, especially triglycerides, which may be a risk factor in coronary heart disease.

Alcohol has a directly poisonous effect on the muscles of the heart. However, alcoholic heart failure occurs only in real alcoholics. In an alcoholic, whose diet is often defective too, the heart beats less forcibly and the person becomes breathless. As the amount of alcohol and the period over which it is drunk increase, so does the damage to the heart: it enlarges and fails. This heart disease is being increasingly recognised as a common and important cause of death of many chronic drinkers.

Coffee

Although a study in America showed that patients who had suffered a heart attack had been consuming more coffee than the average population, there is at present no other evidence that coffee drinking is a factor in the development of coronary heart disease. However, there is some evidence to suggest that coffee may be detrimental to the conducting system in a person suffering from irregularities of heart rhythm, particularly increased heart rate. It is not possible to say whether tea is safer than coffee; what little evidence there is would suggest that of the two, tea is less likely to be harmful. Nobody has done a controlled trial of putting so many people on tea and so many people on coffee and following them up through a number of years. It would, in any case, be virtually impossible to disentangle the different variables which tend to be associated with consumption of tea or coffee—let alone other factors, such as cigarette smoking, heredity, occupation, personality.

Salt

Salt encourages the retention of water in the body. As far as slimming is concerned, cutting down on salt is not going to make any difference to the amount of fat you lose.

However, there is a relationship between salt intake and raised blood pressure, and some suggestion that a high salt intake may play a part in the risk of congestive heart failure. Therefore, it would be a sensible measure for people with raised blood pressure to cut down on salt as far as possible. However, a direct causal relationship between high salt intake and coronary heart disease has not been discovered.

Soft water

The hardness of water—which is a measure of how much calcium and magnesium is dissolved in it (the more, the harder the water)—varies from place to place in the country.

Proportionately more people in soft-water areas die from heart disease than in hard-water areas (studies have looked particularly at men aged 45 to 64). Research has also shown that the death rate from heart disease amongst men of this age has tended to go down where water hardness has increased, and up where it has decreased. In other countries, some studies have—and some have not—supported these findings.

The reason for the lower incidence of heart disease amongst men living in hard-water areas is not understood. One theory is that the trend is a result of hard water not dissolving toxic trace elements, such as lead or cadmium. Until more is known about this, if you use a domestic water softening installation in a hard water area, it is sensible not to include the drinking water.

Oral contraceptives

The increased risk of coronary heart disease from taking oral contraceptives is very slight in a young woman, unless there are other risk factors such as cigarette smoking, raised blood pressure or high level of blood fats.

Any woman should have her blood pressure measured before going on the pill and tell the doctor if there is a family history of coronary heart disease or diabetes or blood fat disorder. The doctor (general practitioner or at the clinic) may send her for a blood test, to find out if she has a raised blood fat content.

There is a statistical correlation between taking oral contraceptives and a rise in blood pressure, and also a small but nevertheless significant increase of risk of coronary heart disease. The risk increases with the length of time that a woman takes the oral contraceptive and also increases after the age of 35 years. After this age, a woman may be well advised to use some other method of contraception, particularly if she is unable to give up cigarette smoking. Younger women, too, would be well advised not to smoke if they use the pill.

Oral contraceptives themselves may lead to raised blood pressure but in the majority of cases the blood pressure returns to normal after stopping the use of the pill. A woman on the pill should make sure to have her blood pressure measured regularly. The pill also carries a small risk of thrombosis in the leg. If the clot then travels to the lungs, this can prove fatal.

To sum up, the use of oral contraceptives increases the risk of coronary heart disease. For a young woman who does not have raised blood pressure this risk is very small. However, it rises with age and probably with protracted use of the pill. The risk is also greatly increased by cigarette smoking because the two causes seem to multiply each other's effect. After the age of 35 the position is more controversial; some people would say the added security against unwanted pregnancy compensates for the extra risk of raised blood pressure or coronary heart disease.

Having a heart attack

What doctors call myocardial infarction or cardiac infarct and the layman calls heart attack occurs when an area of the heart muscle is acutely starved of blood long enough for permanent damage to result.

In some cases, particularly in old people, a heart attack is painless; the person may become confused, breathless, develop swollen ankles. Or the attack may be associated with an abnormality of heart rhythm: the person may be aware of rapid or irregular palpitations—or may not be aware of anything abnormal, depending on what particular arrhythmia is involved. But if and when an electrocardiogram is taken at any later time, this will show up that the person has had a heart attack.

Usually, the major symptom of a myocardial infarction is pain similar in nature to that of angina, but worse. The main difference is that it usually occurs out of the blue and is not brought on by precipitating factors such as effort or emotion (although sometimes it may be associated with effort and emotion). Also, when what seems to be the precipitating cause (exertion or emotion) stops, the pain tends to persist, or persists after taking trinitrin.

The person may collapse, either becoming unconscious or falling to the ground though remaining conscious. Collapsing is one of the words in medicine that means what it says: the person literally collapses.

Giving first aid

Often when somebody collapses in a crowded place, such as a street or railway station or shop, bystanders go to great pains to seem not to have noticed anything amiss. Many people dread finding themselves confronted with a collapsing or collapsed person and having to take positive action, without knowing what to do.

The person administering first aid should have two initial thoughts in mind, and two only: to ensure that the collapsed person's heart is beating adequately, and to ensure that he gets enough air into his lungs. The cause of collapse is very much of secondary importance, and a non-medically qualified person should not try to establish a diagnosis.

Speed is of the essence. First, establish whether the person's heart is beating and whether he is breathing. If neither, begin with mouth-to-mouth resuscitation, quickly followed by heart massage (and then alternate the two). If the heart is beating but the person is not breathing, do mouth-to-mouth resuscitation.

If there is any other person around, make sure that someone phones for an ambulance or in some other way gets medical help.

is the heart beating?

The pulse may be felt on the inside of the wrist about two inches above the base of the thumb. If the heart beat is very weak, the pulse may not be palpable at the wrist, nor if the artery is compressed by the arm lying awkwardly underneath the person's weight. If no pulse can be felt at the wrist, look for, or rather feel for, the carotid pulse, which is situated in the neck and best felt just underneath the angle of the jaw. (Stop reading now and take a moment off to identify these sites on your own body.)

Feel the person's neck; this should be done gently, and certainly not both sides at once for fear of strangling.

Signs of the heart having stopped are a bluish-grey facial colour, dilated pupils and no carotid pulse.

In a very thick-set person with a bull neck or fat neck, the pulse can be difficult to feel. Do not waste time searching. Start emergency resuscitation immediately. Every second counts.

mouth-to-mouth resuscitation

Turn the person's face sideways and clear his mouth of any obstructions—mucus, vomit, false teeth, food. If you feel squeamish about this, cover your hand with a layer of handkerchief. Then turn him on his back and loosen his clothing at the neck and waist. Tilt the head backwards by supporting the nape of the neck and pressing the top of the head; press the chin upwards. This is necessary so that the tongue does not fall to the back of the throat and block the airway.

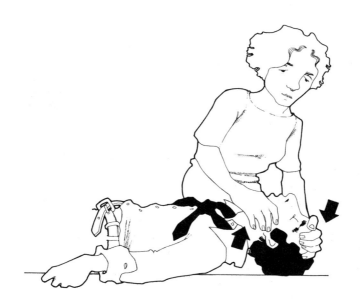

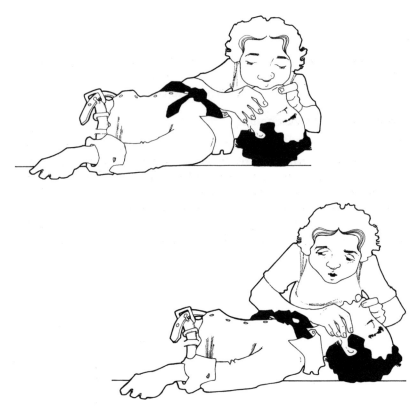

Keep the person's chin lifted up a little with the right hand. Use the finger and thumb of your left hand to pinch together the person's nostrils. (If the nose is not compressed, air blown into the subject's mouth will take the line of least resistance and come out through the nose rather than expand the chest.) Then take a deep breath in, seal your lips round his mouth and blow into his mouth; remove your mouth and watch the chest fall. Repeat, aiming to inflate the lungs approximately once every 5 seconds. Go on doing this, if possible until the subject either starts to breathe spontaneously or a qualified person takes over.

get the heart beating

If no heart beat can be detected, it is reasonable to assume that there is either no heart beat or a grossly inadequate heart beat. In a very fat person this assumption may be wrong, but when you have to make immediate decisions, proceed. A hard sharp thump should be administered to the lower part of the sternum (middle of the chest) with the side of the clenched fist. If this produces an angry response from the person you have thumped, be glad.

Sometimes the thump will start up the heart beat. If not, begin heart massage without delay.

heart massage
If there is no heart beat, heart massage should be started after four mouth-to-mouth inflations.

It is important that the subject should be lying on his back on a hard surface, preferably the floor (a soft bed is quite useless since it is the

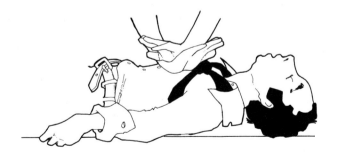

mattress underneath the body which would receive the compression, not the chest itself). The person who administers the massage should kneel beside the body and apply the heel of the right hand over the lower half of the breast bone, and the heel of the other (left) hand across the top of the right hand.

The chest should then be compressed firmly, but not violently, at a rate of about 60 times per minute. You can stop intermittently, to feel for the person's pulse in the hope that the procedure will have started the heart beating on its own. If necessary, the procedure should be continued until medical help arrives.

Cardiac massage is of no value and, in fact, might be dangerous if it is done before mouth-to-mouth resuscitation. Otherwise blood that is made to circulate around the body is not carrying oxygen to the tissues. The blood already in the lungs must be oxygenated before compression forces it through the heart, otherwise chemical damage to the heart muscle can follow.

combined cardiac massage and mouth-to-mouth resuscitation
If there are two people helping the unconscious person, one should administer mouth-to-mouth resuscitation, the other heart massage at about five heart compressions followed by one deep lung inflation. But it is by no means impossible for one person to do both, by alternating massage with inflation of the lungs. A reasonable scheme would be to compress the chest about 5 times, then administer one deep breath, then repeat the process, and so on. This can be quite exhausting and if help is slow to arrive, the limiting factor may not be the patient but the resuscitator's stamina.

A good indication of success is the size of the pupils. Lack of oxygen quickly results in wide dilatation; resuscitation should equally quickly return the pupils to normal size. If they remain widely dilated, either the procedure is not being carried out effectively or the patient has probably suffered from lack of oxygen for too long. The main indication that resuscitation is being effective is that the colour of the face (also of the tongue and inside of lips) changes back from grey/blue to pink.

Quick action

If irreversible damage is to be prevented, resuscitation has to start within 3 to 4 minutes of the heart stopping. The longer it is left, the less the chances of recovery; after about 8 or 9 minutes, there is almost certain to be major brain damage.

Obviously, not everybody who collapses has had a heart attack. There is, after all, such a thing as a simple faint due to sudden sharp drop in blood pressure. However, in such a case the pulse should be readily feelable, even if weak, and the person breathing, although shallowly. So there is no need either for cardiac massage or mouth-to-mouth resuscitation. Loosen the person's collar and belt and raise the legs to about 45 degrees in order to increase the amount of blood returning to the heart, which in turn raises the blood pressure.

Heart failure as against a heart attack is seldom the cause of a sudden collapse, since it usually develops fairly insidiously. But some flooding of the lungs, due to inadequate heart action, may occur quite quickly. In these circumstances, the person's breathing is intensely laboured and noisy, emitting a bubbly sound. He should be propped up in a sitting position. If he becomes unconscious, there is a tendency for him to slide down: make sure he does not do so, by constantly correcting his position while waiting for medical help.

So, to repeat: do not be concerned about subtleties of diagnosis. Just bear in mind the two points: the person should get enough air into his lungs and the heart must be made to beat properly.

Needless to say, having instituted the immediate care of the patient, try to obtain urgent medical help by a 999 call or a doctor if one is to hand. If there is a chance of attracting help either by shouting or literally running out of the door for a few seconds, after having started resuscitation, and shouting to a passer-by or to a neighbour, a really fast sprint of 30 seconds there and back is unlikely to cause irreversible damage. But in a situation where there are no neighbours sufficiently near or no way of attracting help or attention, all you can do is try resuscitation for as long as you reasonably can. Most people find it hard to persevere for more than about 15 minutes from sheer physical exhaustion, and then have to give up.

Fortunately, in most cases the person has in the meantime started breathing again and his heart is beating.

Manuals on first aid are published by the British Red Cross Society and St. John Ambulance; both organisations run first aid courses.

Treatment after a heart attack

People who have a heart attack at work or in the street or in some public place are usually taken by ambulance to the nearest accident and emergency department of a hospital.

Not all heart attacks are so dramatic and unexpected. Often, the person is warned by a gripping pain in the chest, not unlike severe indigestion. Call the doctor immediately and describe your symptoms and ask him to come even if it turns out really to have been no more than indigestion. The majority of people who are going to die after a heart attack do so within the first hour.

home or hospital

The emergency treatment that the general practitioner can carry out at home may be life-saving. It consists of relief of pain, sedation, correction of arrhythmias, if present.

A major role the general practitioner has to play is making the correct diagnosis; a severe chest pain may not necessarily mean a cardiac infarct (although the chest pain from other causes is unlikely to be quite as acute as in a heart attack).

The pain is severe and frightening—and there is a feeling of impending doom. Relief of pain (by the injection of a powerful pain-relieving drug) is the first aspect of emergency treatment. Sedation with a tranquillising drug also helps to relieve the person's acute anxiety.

One of the dangers in a heart attack is the sudden changes in heart rhythm which can result in the circulation virtually stopping. The general practitioner may be able to rectify this with drugs.

The general practitioner must then decide whether to keep the patient at home, or to send him to hospital. Much will depend on the support available in the home, the distance to be travelled to hospital and above all, the patient's previous medical history. Sometimes the general practitioner may call in a specialist (perhaps the hospital's cardiologist) before making the decision—though not in a case of emergency.

ambulance

If the general practitioner is not immediately available (for instance he may be visiting another patient), use the emergency 999 service and get an ambulance to take the patient to a hospital. Getting medical help quickly is more important than getting the help of a particular service. In a large city, you would probably obtain an ambulance more quickly than your general practitioner, in a rural area the reverse is more likely.

The delay between the development of the heart attack and arrival in a coronary care unit cancels out much of the advantage of the specialised facilities available there.

An extensive survey in the UK a few years ago showed that the mean time between development of a heart attack and arrival in the coronary care unit was between 4 and 5 hours. There are various reasons for this, such as that the person does not accept or realise he is having a heart attack and therefore delays in seeking advice and medical help; the medical help does not get there quickly; the ambulance takes time to arrive; there are delays in the process of admission within the hospital.

One important aspect of treatment in the early stages of a heart attack is the alleviation of anxiety. The process of transport to a hospital involves being loaded on and off stretchers and trolleys, a ride in an ambulance, possibly with sirens screaming and lights flashing, all of which is likely to increase the person's anxiety. The ambulance service carry out their duties sympathetically and skillfully. But there may be six flights of stairs to negotiate, thick traffic jams, bad road conditions and a long and awkward drive to the hospital.

In some areas, a coronary care ambulance is available, fully equipped and staffed for resuscitative procedures. The obvious problem is the considerable cost (expensive equipment and highly trained personnel, including doctors).

In Brighton, an experiment has proved successful for some years. Rather than an ambulance designed to cater for coronary care alone, ambulances tailored for most of the common emergencies are available, equipped with the necessary resuscitative gear basic to an intensive care unit or coronary care unit in a hospital. The ambulance men are fully conversant with the relevant life-saving techniques, and trained to recognise and identify arrhythmias, and to give the appropriate treatment. This means that it is not necessary for a doctor to go out in each ambulance. Because the patient is brought to care earlier, there is less likelihood of complications and the hospital stay is therefore likely to be shorter. The ambulances drive at a speed that gives the patient a smooth journey. Because they are fully equipped, speed in reaching the hospital is not necessarily the predominant factor.

Similar special ambulances are in operation in Surrey and some other parts of the country, funded by voluntary contributions. The number of such vehicles is limited.

Coronary care unit

If at the moment of a person having a heart attack he could wave a magic wand and be transported instantaneously into a coronary care unit in hospital, that would be the ideal environment for him, with the best prognosis.

The essential feature of intensive coronary care, as it is sometimes called, is that the care should in fact be intensive. This implies a greater ratio of staff to patients than in other parts of the hospital and usually small units with eight beds or even fewer, with plenty of space around each patient. In the event of an emergency, the personnel involved can have easy access, and bulky apparatus such as an anaesthetic trolley, for instance, can be brought close to the patient. The decor is generally attractive and aimed at creating an atmosphere of tranquillity. The beds are usually positioned or screened in such a way that the patients do not have to see each other.

By each bed is an ECG monitor, oxygen supply, suction supply and an adequate number of electrical sockets in which to plug additional apparatus as and when required; a defibrillator is nearby.

As soon as the patient arrives in the coronary care unit, he is connected to an ECG monitor. The displays on the electrocardiograph are continuously watched by an experienced nurse who is trained to recognise the warning signs. These include increased ectopic activity beyond a certain amount, the development of ventricular tachycardia and the onset of ventricular fibrillation. A major hazard after a heart attack is ventricular fibrillation, a severe irregularity of heart beat. The main reason for intensive monitoring is to detect it, or early warning signs, immediately so that appropriate corrective measures can be applied.

The treatment, known as DC cardioversion, is an electric shock applied to the chest with the help of a defibrillator. A defibrillator is a device capable of administering a DC shock of up to 400 joules from two electrodes which are placed on the patient's chest. They are about three inches in diameter with an insulated handle, something like an upside-down mushroom. The doctor holds the stalk and applies the flat surface to the chest and administers the electric shock. In the majority of cases, the defibrillator will correct ventricular fibrillation and restore a regular heart rhythm. It will not be of any value in cardiac standstill, when there is no electrical activity in the heart whatever. In such a situation, injection of cardiac stimulant drugs is given in order to induce some minimal activity of the heart, to make it amenable to electrical treatment.

immediate coronary care
Generally, the patient is given a morphine type of pain-killer until his chest pain is relieved. He is sedated with a tranquilliser, usually for the first 24 hours, to keep him sleeping lightly but rousable for meals. Drugs to prevent the development of arrhythmias may be given intravenously, or by mouth.

Anti-coagulants may be given (usually subcutaneously) to counteract the risk of venous thrombosis in the leg, or pulmonary embolism, developing.

After 48 hours of complete rest, the patient may be made to undertake hourly leg exercises to prevent thrombosis in the vein of the leg and he is made to do deep-breathing exercises to prevent collapse of the lungs.

Rehabilitation begins when the patient is asked 'What would you like for breakfast?' and starts to make a conscious decision in what happens to him and what is done for him—initially in matters of personal care and hygiene. This progresses as he is allowed more mobility when he is moved from the coronary care unit to the ward.

subsequent care

If there are no problems, the patient is moved from the coronary care unit into the main ward after 2 or 3 days, and is allowed to get out of bed for a short while, progressively longer, and to walk around. In an uncomplicated case, the patient needs to remain in hospital for no longer than about 10 days to a fortnight, unless any complications arise.

Rehabilitation

With discharge from hospital comes the sudden awareness that the human and mechanical monitors, which mean security, are to be removed. This can be quite frightening. The dependence on both medical staff and machines during a cardiac crisis can make people reluctant and afraid to resume responsibility for themselves, particularly when physical ability is still hampered. It is important for the patient to maintain at home the level of independence gained in hospital, and for relatives to encourage him gradually to increase the number of his activities.

The general practitioner has an important role in after-care. He can advise on hours of rest, the type and amount of food to be eaten, and on a programme of graded exercise to be followed, starting with walking.

If you know how far you can walk without distress, halve that distance for your outward journey, because you will have to return to the starting point. When walking out of doors, be aware that extremes of temperature, hot or cold, will reduce the amount of activity you can undertake, and that slopes and hills will reduce the distance possible for you. Such obstacles will have to be attempted gradually, and not accomplished in a day. The doctor or hospital will have discussed the significance of possible distress symptoms such as chest pain, and shortness of breath.

A number of hospitals, aware of the need for a planned return to activity, offer rehabilitation programmes for the patient who has suffered a heart attack. These programmes contain basically two elements: physical activity and a counselling service. They are organised by a variety of personnel; doctors, nurses, physiotherapists, dieticians, occupational therapists and social workers may be involved.

Physical activity

The time spent on physical activities, and their strenuousness, is increased gradually, while breathing and pulse are monitored. In some instances, the patients are taught to monitor themselves. The aim is not olympic fitness, but to achieve as much as is realistic and to regain the quality of life. In most places, the increase in physical activity is organised and supervised by physiotherapists.

Occupational therapists are also becoming more and more involved in the rehabilitation care of heart attack patients. The starting and end point in rehabilitation is decided according to each patient's needs and ability; the activities are graded in complexity and according to how much mobility, strength and concentration they require. The activities done in the occupational therapy department relate to normal daily activities both in the home and at work. Where such facilities are available, the patients spend time in the occupational therapy workshop, undertaking activities for lengthening stretches of time to improve concentration and generally increase work tolerance. Often new activities are offered rather than those familiar to the person, to prevent distress and frustration, because after a heart attack the person's level of concentration and skill may be diminished.

counselling

Counselling may be offered on an individual or group basis. In a group, the sharing of experiences by patients at different stages of rehabilitation can be a great boost. It allows people to verbalise their fears and anxieties, and helps them to adjust to, and accept, their medical condition. One of the aims of the counselling sessions is to dispose of old wives' tales, such as 'you must not raise your arms above your head' or 'from now on, sex is out'.

Sexual activity usually correlates with the physical effort of climbing two flights of stairs. There is no reason why normal sex activities should not be resumed about 5 to 8 weeks after the heart attack (unless the doctor specifically warns you about this) with the familiar partner in familiar circumstances. Orgasmic sexual intercourse raises the blood pressure considerably but such a transient rise has much less importance than, say, driving a car in the rush hour with a lower but more persistent rise in blood pressure. Individuals vary considerably in their need for sex, and the emotional stresses created by a disruption of marital sex can be more harmful to the individual's heart and blood pressure than sex itself.

Reassurance about all these various factors goes together with a steady, if slow, progress in improved physical activity.

The aim of counselling sessions is to give factual information and also to set individual goals for the patient, allowing him to adjust to, and get over the fears associated with, being a 'heart patient'. It is not unusual for men to feel potential eunuchs following a heart attack, not just because of sexual fears but because of unexpressed fears about their occupation being threatened, their damaged image as a husband and a provider, and a sense of having failed—plus anxieties for the future.

the family
Rehabilitation has to include the family and calls for truth and honesty within the family. In some places, counselling extends to a spouses' group, offering information-giving, problem-sorting meetings for patients and their spouses.

It is important that the patient's progress is not hindered by over-protection at home. Just as a child needs to stumble and totter when learning to walk, so the patient needs freedom to increase gradually his physical and social activity.

At the same time, the tendency to use 'I've got a bad heart, I can't do that' as an excuse for no longer carrying out activities he does not like, such as pruning the roses or washing the dishes, should be discouraged. It is better, and less anxiety-making, to admit dislikes than to claim inability to do what is not a very taxing activity.

back to work

After a major heart attack, the patient can expect to be back at work in about 3 months. After a minor one, it could be after 4 weeks. Really hard physical work is unwise; it is usually better to seek lighter work with the same employer than with a different one. In some cases, the general practitioner may be able to help negotiate a return to modified duties or part-time work, before the person resumes his own job.

For some people, a heart attack has a direct effect on their occupation, mainly people involved in heavy labour, working with dangerous machinery or in public transport, such as train drivers. Drivers of public service vehicles and heavy goods vehicles need to inform their employers and their licensing authority and will be banned from using their special driving licence.

The note on an ordinary driving licence that 'You are required by law to inform DVLC Swansea, SA99 1AT at once if you have any disability which is or may become likely to affect your fitness as a driver' means that anyone who has had a heart attack should notify the licensing authority. He should also inform his insurers of the change in medical state, otherwise the insurance cover might be invalid, with all that that implies. Your doctor will advise you when you can start driving again.

Medical aspects of fitness to drive (price £1.40) published by The Medical Commission on Accident Prevention, 50 Old Brompton Road, London SW7 3EA includes a section on all the cardiac conditions which might affect driving ability.

Re-training and resettlement into a new occupation might be arranged with the help of the disablement resettlement officer, who would also be able to give advice, as can the social worker, on the financial implications of early retirement, if this is indicated. But there is no good evidence to show that if a person who has had a heart attack retires altogether, he will live any longer; the boredom and reduced income may well be too heavy a price to pay.

After-effects

A heart attack may leave some permanent residual damage. It usually takes some weeks to find out if recovery is going to be complete or whether some shortness of breath, or angina, will reappear. The risk remains of a further heart attack, also of rhythm disturbances, progressive heart failure and of an embolism from a clot formed in the heart over the scarred muscle. That is why the patient has to have regular follow-up visits.

A hospital check-up about 6 weeks after the onset of the attack usually includes an ECG and X-ray of the heart. It may disclose a need for drug treatment (such as beta-blockers) or, in a few instances, for further tests such as a coronary angiography. But return to work need not await this check-up, especially if the occupation is a light one or the attack was a minor one.

To avoid a further heart attack, the best plan is to identify, if possible, the factors which brought on the first one and then avoid them. The normal life pattern needs to be scrutinised carefully. Usually, the shock and realisation of having sustained and survived a heart attack is sufficient to enable even the most weak-willed to reform. Obviously, cigarette smoking should be absolutely and permanently stopped, work schedules kept within reasonable bounds, responsibility and excess work should be delegated, activities such as walking and swimming included into a regular routine, the diet (and weight) watched and if any of the warning symptoms reappear, let the doctor know straightaway.

However, over-reaction should be avoided: there is no need for the patient to wrap himself in cotton wool in fear and dread of a further attack, convinced he is a thorough cardiac cripple. If sensible measures are adopted, the outlook after a heart attack is good.

Glossary

ADRENAL glands
ductless glands, situated above kidneys, secreting adrenaline and noradrenaline directly into bloodstream

Latin *ad*, at; *renes*, kidneys

ADRENALINE
hormone produced by adrenal glands affecting blood circulation and muscular action

AETIOLOGY
the cause of phenomena, eg of a disease; the science of such causes

Greek *aetia*, cause; *logos*, discourse

ALVEOLI
air sacs of lungs

Latin *alveolus*, small cavity

ANEURYSM
abnormal dilatation of an artery, due to vessel wall yielding and gradually being stretched by pressure of the blood

Greek *aneurusmos*, a widening

ANGINA PECTORIS
condition characterised by constricting pain in the chest, usually radiating to one or both shoulders and arms, caused by transient insufficiency of blood to the heart

Greek *agkhein*, to throttle; Latin *pectus*, chest

ANGIOGRAPHY
rendering blood vessels visible on X-ray film by injecting into them a radio-opaque substance

Greek *aggeion*, vessel; *graphein*, to mark

ANOXIA
state in which body tissues have an inadequate supply of oxygen

Greek *an*, without

AORTA
large artery which leads from left ventricle of the heart and carries blood for distribution to arteries in the body

Greek *aorte*, from *aeiro*, to lift

ARRHYTHMIA
any variation from normal regular rhythm of heart beat

Greek *a*, without; *rhuthmos*, rhythm

ARTERIOGRAPHY
rendering blood vessels visible on X-ray film
by injecting into them a radio-opaque
substance

ARTERIOLE
small branch of artery leading to still smaller
vessels, the capillaries

ARTERIOSCLEROSIS
thickening and hardening of arteries   Greek *arteria*; *scleros*, hard

ARTERIES
blood vessels carrying oxygenated blood from   Greek *arteria*, from *aer*, air; *terein*,
the heart to the tissues of the body, limbs and to keep (in ancient times it was
internal organs   believed that these vessels contained
                                                air)

ATHEROMA
degenerative change (partly fatty) of inner lay- Greek *athare*, porridge
ers of arteries

ATHEROSCLEROSIS
condition characterised by presence of ather-   Greek *athare*, porridge; *scleros*, hard
oma in inner layers of arteries, reducing the
lumen (internal diameter)

ATRIUM
name given to each of the two upper chambers   Latin *atrium*, hall
or cavities of the heart

BETA-BLOCKERS
drugs which paralyse part of the nerves that
operate independently of consciousness, e.g.
those which quicken the heart beat

BRACHIAL
relating to the upper arm   Greek *brakhion*, arm

BRADYCARDIA
slowness of beating of heart (less than 60 beats Greek *bradus*, slow; *kardia*, heart
per minute)

CALORIE
unit of heat. The energy value of food is measured in units of heat called Calories or, strictly speaking, kilocalories. A kilocalorie or Calorie is defined as amount of heat needed to raise temperature of 1 kilogram of water by 1°C

Latin *calor*, heat

CANNULA
tube for insertion into the body

Latin dimunitive of *canna*, reed

CAPILLARIES
minute vessels joining ends of arteries to beginnings of veins

Latin *capillus*, hair

CARDIAC
relating to the heart

Greek *kardia*, heart

CARDIOMYOPATHY
damaged or diseased heart muscle

Greek *kardia*, heart; *mus*, muscle; *pathos*, disease

CARDIOVASCULAR
relating to both heart and blood vessels

Greek *kardia*, heart; Latin *vasculum*, a vessel

CAROTID artery
principal large artery in each side of neck

Greek *karoein*, to stupefy (compression of these arteries being thought to do this)

CATHETER
hollow tubular instrument for passing into cavity in body for investigation or treatment

Greek *kathienai*, to send down

CEREBROVASCULAR
relating to the blood vessels in the brain

Latin *cerebrum*, brain; *vasculum*, a vessel

CLAUDICATION
occurrence of pain due to impairment in the arterial circulation in a limb, usually the leg

Latin *claudicare*, to limp

CONDUCTION
the transmission of excitation through living tissue e.g. through specialised heart muscle fibres

Latin *conducere*, to bring together

CONGESTIVE
refers to the accumulation of fluid in parts of the body, for instance, over-filling of blood vessels

Latin *congerere*, to collect

CORONARY
relating to a vessel or nerve that encircles an organ

Latin *corona*, crown

CORONARY ARTERIES
vessels encircling the heart and supplying it with blood

Latin *corona*, crown

DIAPHRAGM
muscular partition which separates the cavity of the abdomen from that of the chest

Greek *diaphragma*, a partition wall

DIASTOLE
period when ventricles relax and refill with blood in preparation for their next beat

Greek *diastole*, a drawing asunder

ECTOPIC
in an abnormal position

Greek *ektopos*, displaced

ELECTROCARDIOGRAPH
instrument for recording variations in electric currents which occur in heart as it contracts and relaxes

Greek *elektron*, amber, taken as meaning electricity; *kardia*, heart; *graphein*, to mark

ELECTROCARDIOGRAM
record made by an electrocardiograph

Greek *gramma*, a picture

ELECTRODE
electrical terminal

EMBOLISM
obstructing of a small blood vessel by material carried in blood stream; may be a clot or dislodged atheroma which larger vessels had allowed through

Greek *en*, in; *ballein*, to throw

ENDARTERECTOMY
operation in which atheroma is scoured out from inside an artery, or removal of an impacted blood clot

Greek *endon*, within; *arteria*, artery; *aektome*, incision

ENDOCARDITIS
inflammation of membrane lining the heart, especially that over heart valves

Greek *endon*, within; *kardia*, heart

ENDOSCOPE
instrument for examining visually the interior of a hollow organ

Greek *endon*, within; *skopein*, to view

EPIDEMIOLOGY
study of distribution and determinants of disease in populations

Greek *epi*, upon; *demos*, people; *logos*, a discourse

ERGOMETER
instrument for measuring muscular power

Greek *ergon*, work; *metron*, measure

ESSENTIAL HYPERTENSION
raised blood pressure reason for which is unknown

FEMORAL
relating to the thigh

Latin *femur*, thigh

FIBRILLATION
rapid unco-ordinated contractions or tremor of muscles, especially abnormal action of heart muscle

Latin *fibrilla*, dimunitive of *fibra*, fibre

FOCUS
principal seat (of disease, activity, etc)

Latin *focus*, fire-place

HAEMOGLOBIN
oxygen-carrying pigment combined with protein in the red blood cells

Greek *haima*, blood; Latin *globus*, globe

HAEMORRHAGE
any escape of blood from vessels which naturally contain it

Greek *haima*, blood; *rhegnunai*, to break

'HOLE IN THE HEART'
congenital heart disease in which septum does not fully shut off right atrium from left atrium or right ventricle from left ventricle (can be closed surgically by placing a patch over it)

HORMONE
chemical substance secreted by an endocrine gland into blood stream in order to bring about specific changes in distant cells and organs

Greek *horman*, to set in motion

HYPERTENSION
increased tension, especially of arterial system: raised blood pressure

Greek *huper*, over; Latin *tendere*, to stretch

HYPERTROPHY
increase in size of an organ, usually as a result of increased amount of work demanded of it

Greek *huper*, over; *trophe*, nutrition

INCOMPETENT
unable to close properly (of heart valve)

INFARCT(ION)
changes which take place in an organ when an artery becomes obstructed, leading to death of part of organ supplied by the artery

Latin *infarcire*, to stuff into

INTRAVENOUS
into a vein

Latin *intra*, within; *vena*, vein

ISCHAEMIA
bloodlessness of a part of the body due to narrowing or blocking of the arteries supplying that part

Greek *iskhein*, to hold back; *haima*, blood

ISOMETRIC exercise
exercise in which muscles are contracting to hold a fixed or static position irrespective of the resistance, e.g. press-ups

Greek *isos*, equal; *metron*, measure

ISOTONIC exercise
exercise in which muscles are constantly on the move e.g. swimming

Greek *isos*, equal; *tonos*, tone

JOULE
unit of energy or heat (4.2 kilojoules = 1 kilo-calorie)

named after English physicist J. P. Joule 1818–1889

LIPAEMIA
excessive amount of fat in the blood   Greek *lipos*, fat; *haima*, blood

LIPID
fat-like substance   Greek *lipos*, fat

METABOLISM
process of physical and chemical changes by   Greek *metabole*, change
which nutritive material is transformed into
tissues, energy and waste products

MITRAL valve
valve at opening from left atrium into left   Greek *mitra*, head-dress
ventricle of the heart

MYOCARDIAL
relating to muscular tissue of the heart   Greek *mus*, muscle; *kardia*, heart

NICOTINE
poisonous alkaloid extracted as oily liquid   named after J. Nicot, 1530–1600, who
from tobacco   introduced tobacco into France

NORADRENALINE
hormone affecting blood circulation and muscular action, secreted at sympathetic nerve
endings and by adrenal glands

OBESITY
condition of being overweight   Latin *ob*, on account of; *esus*, having
                                                        eaten

OCCLUDE
obstruct, stop up, close off   Latin *ob*; *claudere*, to shut

OEDEMA
abnormal accumulation of fluid in the tissues   Greek *oidema*, a swelling
following its passage through the walls of
vessels

PALPATION
examination by touch   Latin *palpare*, to stroke

PALPITATION
an awareness of the heart beat   Latin *palpitare*, to flutter

PAROXYSM
sudden attack: a sudden increase in the severity of existing symptoms

Greek *para*, beyond; *oxus*, sharp

PLASMA
fluid portion of the blood

Greek *plasma*, from *plassein*, to form

PLATELETS
small blood cells playing an important part in clotting

Greek *platus*, broad

PROGNOSIS
forecast of probable duration, course and outcome of a disease

Greek *pro*, before; *gnosis*, knowledge

PULMONARY
relating to the lungs

Latin *pulmo*, lung

PULMONARY EMBOLISM
blockage of large or small pulmonary artery usually by blood clot

RADIAL
relating to the forearm

Latin *radius*, staff or spoke

REGURGITANT
flowing back (of blood through a defective heart valve)

Latin *regurgitare*, to surge back

RENAL
relating to the kidneys

Latin *renes*, kidney

SAPHENOUS
relating to the two large leg veins

Greek *saphenes*, manifest, visible

SEPTUM
partition between the two sides of the heart

Latin *septum*, wall

SPHYGMOMANOMETER
instrument for measuring arterial blood pressure

Greek *sphugmos*, pulsation; *manos*, thin; *metron*, measure

STENOSIS
unnatural narrowing in any passage or orifice of the body, especially in the four openings of the heart at which valves are situated

Greek *stenos*, narrow

STERNUM
breast-bone

Greek *sternon*, breast

STEROID
group name for compounds with similar chemical structure but widely different actions e.g. cholesterol, sex hormones, cortisone

Greek *stereos*, solid; *eidos*, form

SUBCUTANEOUS
lying or occurring beneath the skin

Latin *sub*, below; *cutis*, skin

SUPRAVENTRICULAR
relating to or arising in atria of the heart

Latin *supra*, above; *ventriculus*, diminutive of *venter*, belly i.e. sac

SYSTOLE
period when ventricles contract and propel blood into the arteries

Greek *sustole*, contraction

TACHYCARDIA
abnormal rapidity of heart's action

Greek *takhus*, swift; *kardia*, heart

THROMBUS
blood clot

Greek *thrombos*, clot

THROMBO-EMBOLISM
blockage of an artery (for instance in the leg) as a result of a piece of thrombus breaking off and being carried along in the blood until it comes to a narrow blood vessel where it causes an obstruction.

Greek *thrombos*, clot; *en*, in; *ballein*, to throw

THROMBOSIS
formation of a blood clot in a blood vessel (coronary thrombosis is formation of a clot in a coronary artery)

Greek *thrombos*, clot

TOXIC

poisonous; caused by poison

Greek *toxikon*, poison

TRICUSPID valve

valve at opening from right atrium into right ventricle of heart

Latin *tres*, three; *cuspis*, a point

VARICOSE

dilated and knotted condition of veins

Latin *varicosus*, from *varix*, a dilated vein

VASCULAR

relating to, consisting of or having vessels

Latin *vasculum*, diminutive of *vas*, a vessel

VASODILATORS

drugs which widen blood vessels thereby improving circulation

Latin *vas*, vessel; *dilatare*, to enlarge

VENA CAVA

each of two large veins (superior and inferior) which lead into right atrium of the heart

Latin *vena*, vein; *cava*, hollow

VENTRICLE

name given to each of the two lower chambers or cavities of the heart

Latin *ventriculus*, diminutive of *venter*, belly i.e. sac

Index

abnormalities of rhythm 25, 26, 27, 28, 34, 85, 89, 97, 99, 100, 107, 111
– treatment 29, 97, 101
adrenaline 16, 17, 43, 50, 73, gl.
ageing 14, 16, 52, 61, 78, 80, 87
alcohol 27, 41, 71, 85
alveoli 10, gl.
ambulance 90, 98, 99
anaemia 22
angina 23, 31, 43 *et seq*, 48, 89, 107, gl.
– false 23
– treatment 44, *et seq*
angiography 34, 46, 107, gl.
ankles, swollen, 22, 24, 40, 42, 89
anti-coagulants 38, 101
anxiety 20, 22, 43, 76, 97, 98, 104
aorta 9, 35, 41, gl.
aortic valve 9, 35, 41
arteries 7, 11, 18, 19, gl.
– coronary 13, 44, 46
atheroma 14, 50, 63, 68, 71, 73, gl.
atherosclerosis 14, 63, 81, gl.
atrial fibrillation 28, 37
atrium 9, 15, 28, 35, 36, gl.
– left 35, 37, 41
– right 13

beta-blockers 29, 45, 65, 107, gl.
blood 7, 9, 10, 11

blood circulation 16, 94
blood clots 37, 38, 39, 48, 51, 63, 88, 107
blood flow 18, 35, 41, 48
blood pressure 7, 18, 20
– controlling 64
– lowering 16, 61, 95
– measuring 19, 20, 24, 31, 61, 66, 87, 88
– raised 18, 19, 20, 32, 40, 49, 61 *et seq*, 80, 82, 86, 105
blood supply 13, 14, 17, 28, 40, 42, 43, 48, 62
– collateral 44, 48
blood test 23, 87
blood vessels 7, 9, 11, 24, 36, 45, 48
– collateral 44, 48
– dilatation 45
– elasticity 18, 35
bradycardia 28, 29, gl.
brain 7, 29, 37, 41, 63
– damage 95
– haemorrhage 63
breathing 9, 10, 92, 95
breathlessness 22, 27, 32, 36, 40, 41, 42, 43, 62, 79, 85, 89, 107
bronchitis 22, 45, 51

Calories 58, 83, gl.
capillaries 7, 9, 10, 36, gl.
carbon dioxide 9, 10

carbon monoxide 11, 50, 52
carboxyhaemoglobin 50. 51
cardiac catheterisation 33, 34
cardiac massage 90, 93, 94, 95
cardiologist 23, 98
cardioversion 101
carotid pulse 90, 91
central nervous system 16
chest pain 22, 32, 43, 79, 97, 101
cholesterol 11, 23, 68 et seq, 73
– level 49, 50, 68, 70, 73
cigarettes 51
– craving for 55
– cutting down 53, 58
– smoke 11, 52
– smoking 44, 49, 50 et seq, 87, 108
clots 37, 38, 39, 48, 51, 63, 88, 107
coffee 27, 85
collapse 89, 95
contraction 15, 16, 18, 26, 27
coronary angiography 34
coronary arteries 13, 34, 46, gl.
– blocked 44
– narrowing 14, 34, 40, 43, 48, 51, 63
coronary bypass 46
coronary care unit 98, 100 et seq.
coronary thrombosis 48
counselling 103, 104, 105

defibrillator 100, 101
dentist 37, 74
diabetes 23, 49, 64, 80, 81, 82, 87
diagnosis 23, 90, 96, 97
diastolic pressure 18, 19, 21, 64, gl.
diet 49, 64, 82, 84, 108
– and cholesterol 69
dietary fibre 84
diuretics 42, 65
dizziness 61
doctor 19, 49, 66
– reporting to 23, 29, 45, 62, 96, 97, 108
driving 72, 77, 107
– licence 106
drugs 29, 68, 80, 97, 101
– antibiotics 37, 38
– anti-coagulants 38, 39, 101
– anti-smoking 55
– beta-blockers 29, 45, 65, 107
– digoxin 42
– diuretics 42, 65
– GTN 44, 45, 89
– hypotensive 64, 65
– painkillers 97, 101
– vasodilators 65, gl.

ECG 24, 26, 31, 32, 73, 89, 100, 107
– portable 25, 31, 74

echocardiography 32, 33
ectopic beats 26, 27, 50, 100, gl.
effort syndrome 22
electrical activation 15, 25, 26, 28, 29
electrocardiogram (*see* ECG) gl.
embolism 37, 39, 48, 63, 101, 107, gl.
emotional stress 16, 17, 22, 27, 31, 43, 45, 46, 49, 57, 64, 66, 72 *et seq*, 105
employer 106
exercise 11, 15, 16, 36, 44, 54, 72, 73, 76, 77, 78, 79, 103
– and angina 43
– test 31, 32
exertion 23, 43, 64, 72, 89

fainting 22, 28, 29, 36, 95
fat 11, 49, 68, 73, 82, 83
– polyunsaturated 69, 70
– saturated 69, 70
fatty acids 69, 73
fibrillation 28, 100, 101, gl.
first aid 89 *et seq*, 96
fluids 32, 36, 41, 62
– retention 24

general practitioner 19, 22, 23, 29, 81, 97, 98, 103, 106

GTN (glyceryl trinitrate) 44, 45

headaches 45, 61
haemoglobin 11, 50, gl.
heart attack 31, 50, 72, 89
– treatment 97 *et seq*
heart beat 15, 24, 26, 29, 42, 90, 93, 94, 96
heart enlargement 23, 24, 36, 85
heart failure 24, 27, 36, 37, 40, *et seq*, 45, 95
– congestive 42, 86
– hypertensive 62
heart-lung machine 38
heart massage 90, 93, 94, 95
heart muscle 22, 26, 29, 40, 48, 51, 85, 89, 94
– thickening 31, 32, 36, 41, 43, 62
heart rate 15, 16, 29
– and beta-blockers 45
– falling 74
– increase 16, 17, 45, 50, 72, 74, 85
heart rhythm abnormalities 25, 26, 27, 28, 33, 85, 89, 97, 99, 100, 107
– treatment 29
heredity 49, 80, 86
hospital 20, 23, 30, 31, 33, 75, 97, *et seq*
hypertension 21, gl. (*see raised blood pressure*)
– essential 62, gl.

indigestion 22, 97
infection 37, 38, 41
ischaemic heart disease 48, 51, gl.
isometric exercises 79, gl.
isotonic exercises 79, gl.

jogging 79

kidneys 7, 41, 62

lungs 7, 9, 10, 36, 41, 42, 88, 90,
    92, 94, 96
– cancer 51
– disease 42, 45
– inflation 92, 94

mitral valve 9, 35, 36, 38, 41, gl.
mouth-to-mouth resuscitation 90,
    91, 92, 94
muscles 7, 11, 15, 16, 17, 22, 54,
    55, 76 (see also heart muscle)
myocardial infarction 48, 89, gl.

nervous system, central 16, 65
– parasympathetic 16, 74
– sympathetic 16, 17, 74
nicotine 50, 51, 52, 53, 55, gl.
noradrenaline 16, 17, 43, 50, 73,
    gl.

obesity 49, 64, 81, 82, gl.
occupational therapist 103, 104

oedema (see swelling) gl.
oral contraceptives 49, 80, 87
organs 16, 17, 41, 42
outpatient 20, 23, 66
oxygen 7, 9, 10, 11, 16, 43, 44,
    45, 51, 94

pacemaker 29, 30
pain 43, 45, 74, 79, 89, 97
– chest 22, 32, 43, 79, 97, 101
painkillers 97, 101
palpitations 22, 45, 61, 89, gl.
– and ectopic beats 26
parasympathetic nerves 16
physiotherapist 103, 104
platelets 11, 51, gl.
postural hypotension 65
potassium 65
pregnancy 52, 62, 88
pulmonary valve 9, 35
– narrowed 42
pulse 15, 19, 24, 90, 95, 104
– carotid 90
pump 7, 19, 28, 35, 40, 41

raised blood pressure 18, 19, 20,
    32, 40, 49, 61 et seq, 80, 82, 86,
    105
– lowering 61
– treatment 64
regurgitant valves (see valves
    incompetent)

rehabilitation 101 *et seq*
relaxation 20, 54, 55, 57, 75, 76
resuscitation 95, 96
– mouth-to-mouth 90, 91, 92, 94, 99
retraining 104, 107
rheumatic heart disease 35, 38
risk 21, 53, 71
risk factors 49, 61, 64, 68, 80
– interaction 49, 64, 68, 75, 81, 82, 87
– women 80, 87

salt 64, 86
sedentary occupation 77
sex 78, 105
side effects 29, 45, 65
slimming 83, 84
smoking 44, 46, 52 *et seq*, 80
– and weight 58
– in pregnancy 52
– stopping 53 *et seq*, 87, 108
– Which? report 60 *(see also cigarettes)*
sphygmomanometer 19, 67, gl.
sport 75, 77, 79
stenosis *(see valves, narrowed)* gl.
stress, emotional 17, 22, 27, 31, 43, 45, 46, 49, 57, 64, 66, 72 *et seq*, 105
– physical 17, 104
stroke 37, 61, 63, 80

sub-acute bacterial endocarditis 37
sugar 71, 83, 84
surgery 34
– for angina 46
– for valve disease 38, 39
swelling 62
– ankles 22, 24, 40, 42, 89
sympathetic nerves 16, 17, 74
symptoms 14, 22, 23, 24, 29, 31, 32, 36, 61, 103, 108
– withdrawal from smoking 55
systolic pressure 18, 19, 20, gl.

tachycardia 27, 100, gl.
thrombosis 48, 88, 101, gl.
thump 93
tricuspid valve 9, 35, 36, gl.
triglycerides 11, 23, 49, 50, 71, 73, 82, 83, 85
trinitrin 44, 89

unconsciousness 22, 29, 89, 95

valves 9
– abnormalities of 32, 34, 36, 37
– and rheumatic fever 38
– aortic 9, 35, 41
– incompetent 34, 36, 37, 41
– mitral 9, 35, 36, 38, 41

– narrowed 34, 35, 37,
38, 41, 42, 43
– pulmonary 9, 35, 42
– surgery 38, 39
– tricuspid 9, 35, 36
veins 7, 9, 42, 45
– varicose 22, gl.
ventricles 9, 15, 29, 36, 41, gl.
– left 18, 40
– right 42

water hardness 86, 87
weight *(see also obesity)*
– excessive 44, 58, 64
– losing 59, 64, 82
work, returning to 106, 107
workaholic 75

X-rays 23, 33, 34, 46, 48, 107

yoga 54, 76

Consumer Publications

Which? way to slim

is the complete guide to losing weight and staying slim. The book separates fact from fallacy, and gives a balanced view of essentials such as suitable weight ranges, target weights, exercise, and the advantages and disadvantages of the different methods of dieting. The book highlights the dangers of being overweight and warns of the risks in middle age, during pregnancy, when giving up smoking. Every aspect of slimming is appraised—from appetite suppressants to yoga.

There are also sections on slimmers' cookery, foods and aids for slimmers, eating out, slimming groups, help from doctors, the psychology of slimming, activity and exercise. Tables of Calorie and carbohydrate values of foods and drinks are provided for easy day-to-day reference.

Pregnancy month by month

tells in detail what can be expected at every stage of antenatal care. The book gives reasons for the various tests and examinations at antenatal clinics, and considers the effects of drugs and food supplements on a pregnant woman and how to deal with the minor ailments that often accompany pregnancy. Sections on genetic counselling, fertility problems, contraception, abortion and provisions for unmarried mothers are also included.

Living through middle age

faces up to the changes that this stage of life may bring, whether inevitable (in skin, hair, eyes, teeth) or avoidable, such as being overweight, smoking or drinking too much, insomnia. It discusses the symptoms and treatment of specific disorders that are fairly common in men and women over 40, and for women the effects of the menopause and gynaecological problems. Psychological difficulties for both men and women are discussed, and the possible need for sexual adjustment. Throughout, practical advice is given on overcoming problems that may arise.

Avoiding back trouble

explains how the spine is constructed and how not to stress it in everyday activities such as housework, driving, lifting and carrying, gardening, sitting. It describes symptoms of back trouble and advises on how to cope with an acute attack of back pain. It tells what to expect when examined by specialists (including the diagnostic terms that may be used) and the treatments that may be prescribed. The book ends with suggestions about how to avoid becoming a chronic back sufferer.

Having an operation

describes the procedure for admission to hospital and tells you what happens there: ward routine, hospital personnel, preparation for the operation, anaesthesia, post-operative treatment and recovery, arrangements for discharge, and convalescence. Basic information is given about some of the more common operations.

The newborn baby

deals primarily with the first weeks after the baby is born, with information about feeding and development in the following weeks and months. The daily routines, such as feeding, bathing, nappy changing, sleeping, are covered and the book tells how to identify and cope with minor upsets that may cause alarm but are normal and also the more serious ailments that should be reported to the doctor. The book also deals with routine matters such as immunisation, tests, visits to the clinic.

Treatment and care in mental illness
deals briefly with the illnesses concerned and describes the help available through the national health service, from the local authority and from voluntary organisations. It explains the medical treatment a mentally ill person receives as an outpatient or an inpatient, and deals with community care and aftercare. It includes a chapter on the symptoms and treatment of mental illness in old age.

On getting divorced
explains the procedure for getting a divorce in England or Wales, and how, in a straightforward undefended case, it can be done by the postal procedure and without paying for a solicitor. The legal advice scheme and other state help for someone with a low income is described, and there is advice on coping with the home and children in reduced circumstances. Calculations for maintenance and division of property are given with details of the orders the court may make for financial settlements between the divorcing couple and for arrangements about the children.

Where to live after retirement
tackles the difficult subject of a suitable place to live in old age. The book offers practical advice on the decision whether to move or to stay put and adapt the present home to be easier to live in. It weighs up the pros and cons of the alternatives open to an older person, and

the financial aspects involved, considers sheltered housing and granny flats, the problems of living in someone else's household, and residential homes.

The Good Food Guide
published annually in March, the Guide includes restaurants, hotels, pubs and wine bars all over the British Isles and Ireland, assessed from individual reports and independent inspections. The GFG is outspoken, and gives a clear description of the eating places (with details of opening times and all-in prices) so that you can judge for yourself the character, quality and cost of a place before you go there, and can avoid expensive mistakes.

The Good Food Guide Dinner Party Books
contain recipes from chefs and owners of restaurants in *The Good Food Guide*. The recipes in the two books are arranged so that you can plan appropriate and interesting seasonal meals. Ingredients and instructions are complemented by tips about alternatives, preparation, timing and serving, and wines.

The Buyer's Right
provides background information to help you make wise buying decisions and get the best from the money you spend on goods and services. The book offers advice on managing your money and budgeting; deciding on what you need and how best to meet those requirements; choosing between brands; whether to pay by cash or credit and where to go for the best deal.

The Which? Book of House Plants
is a practical guide to choosing, buying and caring for your house

plants. Part one covers looking after your plants, part two gives details and full colour pictures of plants, and part three features the best ways to arrange and display your house plants. Each plant genus is described in detail, with advice on buying, how it reacts to different light, temperature and humidity, watering and feeding, how to propagate new stock and avoid common disorders. The plants are arranged alphabetically in groups of plant types, and indexed with cross-references to colloquial and botanical names.

Earning money at home
is for the person who has to stay at home, and would like to make some money at the same time. The book explains what this entails in the way of organising domestic life, family and children, keeping accounts, taking out insurance, coping with tax, costing, dealing with customers, getting supplies. It suggests many activities that could be undertaken, with or without previous experience.

Dismissal, redundancy and job hunting
for anyone who has been made redundant or dismissed unfairly, the book explains the relevant legislation, minimum payments to which you may be entitled, how you can take your case to an industrial tribunal, how to claim unemployment benefit, what re-training opportunities there are, and how to set about looking for—and finding—another job.

Wills and probate
stresses the advisability of making a will, explains how to prepare one, sign it and have it witnessed. It gives examples of different types of wills showing consideration for the effects of capital transfer tax. The section about probate deals in detail with the administration of

an estate without a solicitor, and illustrates the various situations and problems that might arise.

What to do when someone dies

deals with the procedures that have to be followed after a death: getting the doctor's certificate, registering the death, obtaining death certificates, reporting a death to the coroner and what this entails, arranging for a burial or cremation and the funeral. A final section covers the national insurance benefits to be claimed.

Which? way to buy, sell and move house

takes you through all the stages of moving to another home: house hunting, viewing, estimating costs, having a survey, making an offer, getting a mortgage, completing, selling the present home. Practical arrangements for the move and any necessary repairs to the new home are dealt with, and advice is given on packing and moving possessions, with a removal firm or on your own, and on the day of the move.

The legal side of buying a house

covers the procedure for buying an owner-occupied house with a registered title in England or Wales (not Scotland) and describes the part played by the solicitors and building society, the estate agent, surveyor, Land Registry, insurance company and local authority. It takes the reader step by step through a typical house purchase so that, in many cases, he can do his own conveyancing without a solicitor; it also deals with the legal side of selling.

Extending your house

describes what is involved in having an extension built on to a house or bungalow, explaining what has to be done, when and by whom. It explains how the Building Regulations affect the position and design of an extension, and how to apply for planning permission and Building Regulations approval.

Central heating

helps you to choose central heating for your home, tells you how to find a good installer to carry out the work and gives details of the equipment involved. The book discusses the merits of the different fuels and helps you assess their relative running costs. It highlights the importance of improving insulation, to keep the heat in. There is a section dealing with problems and hazards that might arise after installation.

Cutting your cost of living

helps you take care of the pence—and the pounds, too. It advises you on how to cut down your spending by adapting your shopping habits, how to make small savings (on food, heating, gardening) and larger ones (on travel, do-it-yourself, holidays, luxuries), giving warnings about false economies and guidance on how to take advantage of what is available free.

Consumer Publications are available from
Consumers' Association, Caxton Hill, Hertford SG13 7LZ
and from booksellers.